ethics

in Obstetrics and Gynecology

Second Edition

The American College of
Obstetricians and Gynecologists
Women's Health Care Physicians

409 12TH STREET, SW
PO BOX 96920
WASHINGTON, DC 20090-6920

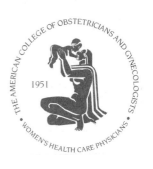

D1299688

Ethics in Obstetrics and Gynecology was developed by the ACOG Committee on Ethics (2003–2004)

Arlene J. Morales, MD, Chair
Carol W. Saffold, MD, Vice Chair
Judith Bernstein, RNC, PhD
Jeffrey L. Ecker, MD
Robert P. Lorenz, MD

Anne Drapkin Lyerly, MD
Daniel J. Martin, Sr, MD
Carl Morton, MD
Carol A. Tauer, PhD
Robert S. Wachbroit, PhD

Jeffrey R. Botkin, MD, Liaison, American Academy of Pediatrics
Monique A. Spillman, MD, PhD, Liaison, American Medical Association
    Council on Ethical and Judicial Affairs
Lorna A. Marshall, MD, Liaison, American Society for Reproductive Medicine

Stanley Zinberg, MD, MS, Vice President, Practice Activities
Mary F. Mitchell, Director, Professionalism and Gynecologic Practice
Megan McReynolds, Project Associate
Lyndona Charles, Special Assistant

Library of Congress Cataloging-in-Publication Data

Ethics in obstetrics and gynecology / the American College of
Obstetricians and Gynecologists.—2nd ed.
    p. ; cm.
Includes bibliographical references and index.
  ISBN 1-932328-03-3
  1. Gynecology—Moral and ethical aspects. 2. Obstetrics—Moral and
ethical aspects.
  [DNLM: 1. Obstetrics—ethics. 2. Ethics, Research. 3.
Gynecology—ethics. 4. Patient Rights—ethics. 5. Reproductive
Techniques—ethics. WQ 21 E844 2004] I. American College of
Obstetricians and Gynecologists.

  RG103.E87 2004
  174.2'982—dc22

                        2003019606

Copies of *Ethics in Obstetrics and Gynecology* can be ordered through the ACOG
Distribution Center by calling toll free 800-762-2264. Orders also can be placed from
the ACOG web site at www.acog.org or sales.acog.org.

12345/87654

DEDICATION

In memory of Kenneth J. Ryan, MD, former chair of the Committee on Ethics
of the American College of Obstetricians and Gynecologists
and the Ethics Committee of the American Society for Reproductive Medicine.
Dr. Ryan brought ethics and ethical decision making to the forefront
of the activities of the American College of Obstetricians and Gynecologists.
His influence then and his legacy for the future will serve to
remind us all of the ethical obligations we must follow
in the day-to-day dealings with our patients, our society, and ourselves.

CONTENTS

PREFACE

The purpose of the second edition of *Ethics in Obstetrics and Gynecology* is to help obstetrician–gynecologists understand and apply the concepts of biomedical ethics to problems in clinical practice, research, and the provision of health care in the community. As the chapters reflect, these professional areas frequently intersect. However, for ease of use, this edition has been reorganized so that related ethical obligations are grouped together. Part I, "Ethical Foundations," describes various theoretical approaches to ethical decision making, offers a stepwise guideline for decision making, addresses common issues faced in daily practice, and offers detailed information on the rationale for obtaining the informed consent of patients and practical assistance as to how this is done. Part II, "Caring for Patients," provides ethical guidance for obstetrician–gynecologists in providing specific health services to their patients. Part III, "Professional Responsibilities," speaks to the ethical obligations that arise out of obstetrician–gynecologists' nonclinical duties as students, teachers, and researchers. This part also identifies appropriate interactions with patients expected as a part of professional behavior. Part IV, "Societal Responsibilities," addresses the ethical obligations of obstetrician–gynecologists to society.

This edition of *Ethics in Obstetrics and Gynecology* adds the following new chapters originally published in 2002 and 2003 as Committee Opinions issued by the Committee on Ethics of the American College of Obstetricians and Gynecologists (ACOG):

- Patents, Medicine, and the Interests of Patients (originally published with ACOG's Committee on Genetics as "Patents, Medicine, and the Interests of Patients: Applying General Principles to Gene Patenting," No. 277, November 2002)

- Research Involving Women (originally published as "Ethical Considerations in Research Involving Women," No. 290, November 2003)
- Surgery and Patient Choice (originally published as "Surgery and Patient Choice: The Ethics of Decision Making," No. 289, November 2003)

Substantial changes to the content have been made to the following chapters for this edition:

- In Part I: Informed Consent
- In Part II: Human Immunodeficiency Virus; Patient Choice in the Maternal–Fetal Relationship; Sex Selection; Multifetal Pregnancy Reduction; Adoption; Sterilization of Women, Including Those With Mental Disabilities; End-of-Life Decision Making
- In Part III: Obstetric–Gynecologic Education
- In Part IV: Relationships With Industry; Expert Testimony

Readers should note that the following chapters from the first edition have been withdrawn because they are no longer current and no longer reflect ACOG policy:

- Endorsement of Institutional Ethics Committees
- Physician Responsibility Under Managed Care: Patient Advocacy in a Changing Health Care Environment

Ethics in Obstetrics and Gynecology also includes the revised "Code of Professional Ethics of the American College of Obstetricians and Gynecologists," issued January 2004. It is an excellent guide for the specialty of obstetrics and gynecology and appears in the appendix.

The Committee on Ethics wishes to acknowledge the assistance of Michael K. Lindsay, MD, for writing the chapter "Research Involving Women" and his previous leadership of the committee.

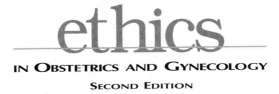

ethics

IN OBSTETRICS AND GYNECOLOGY

SECOND EDITION

PART I
Ethical Foundations

"Good individual decision making encompasses three elements: self-knowledge, knowledge of moral theories and traditions, and cultural perception."—*Encyclopedia of Bioethics*

Because the moral development of the obstetrician–gynecologist as a health care professional begins at the undergraduate level, the Association of Professors in Gynecology and Obstetrics has recommended that ethical principles and concepts be addressed early in career development, as a part of the obstetric–gynecologic clerkship. This core competency is further developed as the obstetrician–gynecologist enters residency training. The Council on Resident Education in Obstetrics and Gynecology and the Accreditation Council on Graduate Medical Education specify the inclusion of training in bioethics as a part of the obstetric–gynecologic residency program, and the American Board of Obstetrics and Gynecology, Inc, examines candidates for board certification on ethical problems in gynecology and obstetrics.

This part of Ethics in Obstetrics and Gynecology *supports the undergraduate and graduate medical education obstetrician–gynecologists receive and aims to encourage and facilitate their lifelong learning in bioethics. It describes leading approaches to bioethical thought, outlines a process for ethical decision making in obstetrics and gynecology, and explains the development and practice of the ethical concept of informed consent.*

1

Ethical Decision Making in Obstetrics and Gynecology

The importance of ethics as applied to the practice of medicine was manifested at least 2,500 years ago in the Hippocratic tradition, which emphasized the virtues that were expected to characterize and guide the behavior of physicians. In the last half of the 20th century, medical technology expanded exponentially, so that obstetrician–gynecologists face complex ethical questions, such as those related to assisted reproductive technologies, prenatal diagnosis and selective abortion, medical care at the beginning and end of life, and the use of genetic information. These problems cannot be solved with medical knowledge alone. Responsible decisions in these areas depend on a thoughtful consideration of the values, interests, rights, goals, and obligations of those involved, all of which are the concern of medical ethics. The formal discipline of biomedical ethics and structured analysis can facilitate the resolution of ethical problems.

Knowledge of ethics and sensitivity toward ethical issues varies widely among physicians. It is important for physicians to improve their skills in addressing ethical decisions through formal undergraduate and graduate medical education, organized continuing education, or personal experience and reading.

Theoretical Background for Ethical Decision Making

Overview of Leading Approaches

In recent decades, medical ethics has been dominated by principle-based ethics (1, 2). In this approach, 4 principles offer a systematic and relatively objective way to identify, analyze, and address ethical dilemmas: 1) respect for patient autonomy, 2) beneficence, 3) nonmaleficence, and 4) justice. Critics of principle-based ethics claim that many difficult clinical problems cannot be adequately resolved or even helpfully evaluated using a principle-based approach. Several alternative approaches have been promoted: virtue-based ethics, care ethics, feminist ethics, communitarian ethics, and case-based reasoning, all of which have merit as well as limitations (3–8).

Virtue-based ethics relies on health professionals' possessing those qualities of character that dispose them to make choices and decisions that achieve the well-being of patients. These qualities of character include trustworthiness, prudence, fairness, fortitude, temperance, integrity, self-effacement, and compassion. Virtues do not replace principles as a basis for ethical behavior or ethical decision making; they enhance and complement the principles of medical ethics. Interpreting the principles, applying them in concrete situations, and setting priorities among them requires the moral sensitivity and judgment of an individual of good character or a virtuous individual.

Care ethics focuses on the character traits that individuals value deeply in close personal relationships, such as sympathy, compassion, fidelity, love, and friendship. This approach downplays the role of rights and allegedly universal principles and suggests that good decisions result from personal caring and interpersonal relations.

Feminist ethics focuses on the experiences of women, rethinking traditional ethics for whatever male bias it may contain. Ethical decisions involving women's health care may be biased by attitudes and traditions about gender roles that are embedded in our culture. Feminist ethics challenges these presuppositions and their consequences. Although similar to care ethics in that it emphasizes the caring virtues, feminist ethics stresses the equality of women and men and the right of women to equal consideration and just treatment. There is evidence that women have been systematically neglected in health care research, financing, and policy making (9–11). Women's health care by its very nature should reflect the concerns from which feminist ethics evolved.

Communitarian ethics challenges the primacy often attributed to personal autonomy in principle-based ethics. It emphasizes the shared values, ideals, and goals of the community and suggests that the needs of the larger community may take precedence, in some cases, over the rights and desires of individuals.

Case-based reasoning is ethical decision making based on precedents set in specific cases, analogous to the role of case law in jurisprudence. An accumulated body of influential cases and their interpretation provide moral guidance. Case-based reasoning asserts the priority of practice over theory and rejects the primacy of moral principles. It recognizes the principles that emerge by a process of generalization from the analysis of cases but views these principles as always open to future revision.

Enlightened ethical decision making in clinical medicine cannot rely exclusively on any single fundamental approach to biomedical ethics. Clinical problems often are too complex to be resolved with simple rules or a rigid application of ethical principles. It is virtues such as prudence, fairness, and trustworthiness that enable the ethical principles to be applied effectively in situations in which there is a conflict of principles or moral values. The specific virtues that are emphasized may vary from one circumstance to another, but in women's health care, there must be particular sensitivity to the needs of women. Furthermore, in almost every difficult situation requiring ethical insight, there is tension between the well-being and interests of the individual patient and the interest of the "community," however that is defined. Finally, no good ethical decision is made without awareness of and guidance from how such decisions have been made in the past. A principle-based approach is a reasonable basis for ethical decision making provided that it incorporates the valuable contributions and insights of alternative approaches to ethical problems.

Ethical Principles

The major principles that are commonly invoked as guides to professional action and for resolving conflicting obligations in health care are respect for autonomy, beneficence and nonmaleficence, and justice (2). Other principles also may be important, such as fidelity.

Autonomy. Autonomy derives from the Greek autos ("self") and nomos ("rule" or "governance") and literally means self-rule. In medical practice, the principle of autonomy implies personal rule of the self that is free both from controlling interferences by others and from personal limitations that prevent meaningful choice, such as inadequate understanding (2). Respect for a patient's autonomy acknowledges an individual's right to hold views, to make choices, and to take actions based on personal values and beliefs. Autonomy provides a strong moral foundation for informed consent, in which a patient, fully informed about her medical condition and the available therapies, freely chooses to be a willing participant in any treatment or nontreatment. Respect for patient autonomy, like all ethical principles, cannot be regarded as absolute and may at times be in conflict with other principles or other moral considerations.

Beneficence and Nonmaleficence. Beneficence, which literally means doing or producing good, is the obligation to promote the well-being of others. It is the principle requiring that a physician must act in a manner that benefits the patient. Nonmaleficence is the obligation not to harm or cause injury and is best known in the maxim primum non nocere: "First, do no harm." Although there are some subtle distinctions between nonmaleficence and beneficence, they often are considered as manifestations of a single principle. These 2 principles taken together are operative in almost every decision to treat patients, because every medical or surgical treatment has both benefits and risks, which must be balanced knowledgeably. Beneficence, the obligation to promote the well-being of the patient, may be in conflict with the need to respect the patient's autonomy. For example, a patient may desire to deliver a fatally malformed fetus by cesarean because she believes that this procedure will increase the chance of the newborn surviving, if only for a few hours. The physician's best judgment is that the risks to the woman of the surgical delivery do not justify the theoretical benefit to a "nonviable" infant. In such a situation, the difficulty of the physician's task is compounded by having to consider the patient's psychologic, physical, and spiritual well-being.

Justice. Justice is the principle of rendering what is due to others. It is the most complex of the ethical principles to be considered because it deals not only with the physician's obligation to render to a patient what is owed but also with the physician's role in the allocation of limited medical resources in the community. Also, there are various means of determining what is owed and to whom it is owed using criteria such as need, effort, contribution, or merit. Justice is the obligation to treat equally those who are alike or similar according to whatever criteria are selected. Individuals should receive equal treatment unless it is demonstrated that they differ from others in ways that are based on science and relevant to the treatments in question. Determination of the criteria on which these judgments are based is a moral decision and is highly complex, as exemplified by ethical controversies about providing or withholding renal dialysis and organ transplantation.

The principle of justice applies at many levels. At the societal level, it addresses the criteria for allocating scarce resources, such as organs for transplantation. At a more local level, it is relevant to questions such as which patients (and physicians) receive priority for operating room times. Even at the level of the physician–patient relationship, the principle of justice applies to matters such as the timing of patient discharge. The principle also governs relationships between physicians and third parties, such as payors and regulators. In the context of the physician–patient relationship, the physician should be the patient's advocate when institutional decisions about allocation of resources must be made.

Guidelines for Decision Making

Often, more than 1 course of action may be morally justifiable. At times, no course of action will seem acceptable, because each may result in significant harms. Nevertheless, one of the available options must be selected and its choice supported with ethical reasoning. Attempts to resolve such difficulties can be aided by a rational analysis of the various factors involved. In addition, the involvement of individuals with a variety of backgrounds and perspectives can be useful when ethical questions are being addressed. Consultation with those from related services or with a hospital ethics committee can be very helpful in ensuring that all viewpoints and possibilities are considered as a decision is made.

It is important for the individual physician to develop a decision-making scheme that can be consistently applied when ethical dilemmas are faced. An approach consisting of logical steps can aid the practitioner in approaching an ethical problem.

Several useful schemes have been proposed (12–15), elements of which are incorporated here.

1. *Identify the decision makers.* The first step in addressing any problem is to answer the question "Whose decision is it?" Generally, the patient is presumed to have the authority and capacity to choose among medically acceptable alternatives or to refuse treatment.

   a. At times, the patient's ability to make a decision is not clear. An individual's capacity to make a decision depends on that individual's ability to understand information and appreciate the implications of that information when making a personal decision (16). In contrast, competence and incompetence are legal determinations that may or may not truly reflect functional capacity. Assessment of a patient's capacity to make decisions must at times be made by professionals with expertise in making such determinations. Decisions about competence can be made only in a court of law.

   b. If a patient is thought to be incapable of making a decision or has been found legally incompetent, a surrogate decision maker must be identified. In the absence of a durable power of attorney, family members have been called on to render proxy decisions. In some situations, the court may be called on to appoint a guardian. A surrogate decision maker should make the decision that the patient would have wanted or, if the patient's wishes are not known, that will promote the best interests of the patient. The physician has an obligation to assist those representing the patient in examining the issues and reaching a resolution.

   c. In the obstetric setting, a pregnant woman generally is considered the appropriate decision maker for the fetus that she is carrying.

2. *Collect data, establish facts.*

   a. It is important to be aware that perceptions about what may or may not be relevant or important to a case are based on personal values. One should remain as objective as possible when collecting the information on which a decision will be based.

   b. Use consultants as needed to ensure that all available information about the diagnosis, treatment, and prognosis has been obtained.

3. *Identify all medically appropriate options.*

   a. Use consultation as necessary.

   b. Identify other options raised by the patient or other concerned parties.

4. *Evaluate options according to the values and principles involved.*

   a. Start by gathering information about the values of the involved parties, and try to get a sense of the perspective and values each is bringing to the discussion. The values of the decision maker will be the most important as decision making proceeds.

   b. Decide whether any of the options violates ethical principles that all agree are important. Eliminate those options that, after analysis, are found to be morally unacceptable by all parties.

   c. Reexamine the remaining options according to the interests and values of each party. Some alternatives may be successfully combined.

5. *Identify ethical conflicts and try to set priorities.*

   a. Try to define the problem in terms of the ethical principles involved (eg, beneficence versus autonomy).

   b. Weigh the principles underlying each of the arguments made. Does one of the principles appear more important than others as the conflict is examined? Does one proposed course of action seem to have more merit than the others?

   c. Consider respected opinions about similar cases and decide to what extent they can be useful in addressing the current problem. Look for morally relevant differences and similarities between this and other cases. Usually, it will be found that the basic dilemma at hand is not a new one and that points considered by others in resolving past dilemmas can be useful.

6. *Select the option that can be best justified.* Try to arrive at a rational resolution to the problem, one that can be justified to others in terms of ethical principles with universal appeal.

7. *Reevaluate the decision after it is acted on.* Repeat the evaluation of the major options in light of information gained during the implementation of the decision. Was the best possible decision made? What lessons can be learned from the discussion and resolution of the problem?

Common Problems in Ethical Decision Making

Although almost everything obstetrician–gynecologists do in their professional lives involves 1 or more of the ethical principles and the personal virtues to a greater or lesser degree, there are several specific areas that deserve special attention: the role of the obstetrician–gynecologist in the society at large, the process of informed consent, confidentiality, and conflict of interest.

The Obstetrician–Gynecologist's Role in Society at Large

In addition to their ethical responsibilities in direct patient care, obstetrician–gynecologists have ethical responsibilities related to their involvement in the organization, administration, and evaluation of health care. This responsibility is exercised through membership in professional organizations; consultation with and advice to community leaders, government officials, and members of the judiciary; expert witness testimony; and education of the public. Justice is both the operative principle and the defining virtue in decisions about the distribution of scarce health care resources and the provision of health care for the medically indigent and uninsured. The virtues of truth telling, fidelity, trustworthiness, and integrity must guide physicians in their roles as expert witnesses, as consultants to public officials, and as educators of the lay public (see "Expert Testimony" in Part IV).

Informed Consent Process

Informed consent is "the willing and uncoerced acceptance of a medical intervention by a patient after adequate disclosure by the physician of the nature of the intervention, its risks and benefits, as well as of alternatives with their risks and benefits" (13). The primary purpose of the consent process is the protection of patient autonomy. By encouraging an ongoing and open communication of relevant information (full disclosure), the physician enables the patient to exercise personal choice. This sort of communication is central to an appropriate physician–patient relationship. Unfortunately, discussions for the purpose of educating and informing patients about their health care options are never completely free of the informant's bias. Practitioners should attempt to be aware of their own biases and make an effort to maintain objectivity in the face of those biases, while disclosing to the patient personal biases that may influence the practitioner's recommendations (17, 18). A patient's right to make her own decisions about medical issues extends to the right to refuse recommended medical treatment. Freedom to accept or refuse recommended medical treatment is supported legally as well as ethically.

One of the most important elements of informed consent is the patient's capacity to understand the nature of her condition and the benefits and risks of the treatment that is recommended as well as those of the alternative treatments. A patient's capacity to understand depends on her maturity, state of consciousness, mental acuity, education, cultural background, native language, the opportunity and willingness to ask questions, and the way in which the information is presented. Diminished capacity to understand is not necessarily the same as legal incompetence. Psychiatric consultation may be helpful in establishing a patient's capacity, or ability to comprehend information that is provided. Critical to the process of informing the patient is the physician's integrity in choosing the information that is given to the patient and respectfulness in presenting it in a manner in which it can be comprehended. An important element of informed consent is the concept of voluntariness—the patient's freedom to choose among alternatives. Informed consent should be free from coercion, pressure, or undue influence (see "Informed Consent" in Part I).

Confidentiality

Confidentiality applies when an individual to whom information is disclosed is obligated not to divulge this information to a third party. Rules of confidentiality are among the most ancient components of codes of medical ethics. Confidentiality is based on the principle of patient autonomy, which includes a patient's right to privacy and the physician's fidelity-based responsibility to respect a patient's privacy. Assurance of confidentiality allows patients to disclose information that may be essential in making an accurate diagnosis and planning appropriate treatment. There are, however, legal exceptions to confidentiality, such as the requirements for reporting certain sexually transmitted diseases or suspected child abuse. The need for storing and transmitting medical information about patients is a serious threat to confidentiality, a problem made more complex by the use of electronic storage and transmission of patient data. The recent increase in the use of genetic testing and screening also emphasizes the need for confidentiality and patient privacy, because genetic information has lifelong implications for patients and their families.

Obstetrician–gynecologists are confronted with issues of confidentiality in dealing with adolescents, especially regarding the diagnosis and treatment of sexually transmitted diseases, contraceptive counseling, and pregnancy (19). The physician's willingness and ability to protect confidentiality should be discussed with all adolescent patients early in their care. Many state laws protect adolescent confidentiality in certain types of situations, and obstetrician–gynecologists should be aware of the laws in their own states.

Conflict of Interest

Conflicts of interest occur almost daily in any obstetrician–gynecologist's practice. A conflict of interest occurs when a primary interest (usually the patient's well-being) is in conflict with a secondary interest (such as, the physician's financial interest). Some conflicts are very obvious as when managed care guidelines limit coverage for diagnostic testing that physicians consider necessary for patients or when physicians recommend products to patients that are sold for a profit in their offices (see "Commercial Enterprises in Medical Practice" in Part III). Some conflicts of interest are subtle as in referral of patients for tests or procedures to an entity in which the physician has a financial interest or attending a continuing education event sponsored by a drug or equipment manufacturing company. Contributions from industry may create a conflict of interest.

There is ever-increasing intrusion into the patient–physician relationship by government and the marketplace. Care plans, practice guidelines, and treatment protocols may substantially limit physicians' ability to provide what they consider proper care for patients. Incentive plans may create inducements to limit care in the interest of increasing physicians' incomes. Whereas at one time, the tension between physicians' financial self-interest and patients' interests often encouraged unnecessary testing and too much treatment, the current tension may provide incentives for too little care. Conflicts of interest should be avoided whenever possible, and when they are material and cannot be avoided, it is the physician's responsibility to disclose them to patients.

Summary

Obstetrician–gynecologists who are familiar with the concepts of medical ethics will be better able to approach complex ethical situations in a logical and organized fashion. They will understand that patients' personal goals and values affect their choices and thereby influence clinical decisions. By consulting the ethical frameworks provided by principles, virtues, caring and feminist perspective, concern for community, and case precedents, they will enhance their ability to make clinical decisions that respect the values and promote the best interests of patients.

References

1. Ross WD. The right & the good. Indianapolis (IN): Hackett Publishing Company; 1988.
2. Beauchamp TL, Childress JF. Principles of biomedical ethics. 5th ed. New York (NY): Oxford University Press; 2001.
3. Steinbock B, Arras JD, London AJ. Ethical issues in modern medicine. 6th ed. Boston (MA): McGraw Hill; 2003.
4. Beauchamp TL, Walters L. Contemporary issues in bioethics. 6th ed. Belmont (CA): Wadsworth Publishing; 2003.
5. Mappes TA, DeGrazia D. Biomedical ethics. 5th ed. Boston (MA): McGraw-Hill; 2001.
6. McCullough LB, Chervenak FA. Ethics in obstetrics and gynecology. New York (NY): Oxford University Press; 1994.
7. Pellegrino ED. The metamorphoses of medical ethics. A 30-year retrospective. JAMA 1993;269:1158–62.
8. Pellegrino ED, Thomasma DC. The virtues in medical practice. New York (NY): Oxford University Press; 1993.
9. Merkatz RB, Temple R, Subel S, Feiden K, Kessler DA. Women in clinical trials of new drugs. A change in Food and Drug Administration policy. The Working Group on Women in Clinical Trials. N Engl J Med 1993;329:292–6.
10. Weisman CS. Women's health care: activist traditions and institutional change. Baltimore (MD): Johns Hopkins University Press; 1998.
11. Gender disparities in clinical decision making. Council on Ethical and Judicial Affairs, American Medical Association. JAMA 1991;266:559–62.
12. Pellegrino ED. The anatomy of clinical-ethical judgments in perinatology and neonatology: a substantive and procedural framework. Semin Perinatol 1987;11:202–9.
13. Jonsen AR, Siegler M, Winslade WJ. Clinical ethics: a practical approach to ethical decisions in clinical medicine. 4th ed. New York (NY): McGraw-Hill; 1998.
14. Kanoti GA. Ethics and medical–ethical decisions. Crit Care Clin 1986;2:3–12.
15. Abrams FR. Bioethical considerations for high-risk pregnancy. In: Abrams RS, Wexler P, editors. Medical care of the pregnant patient. Boston (MA): Little, Brown and Co; 1983. p. 1–12.
16. Grisso T, Appelbaum PS. Assessing competence to consent to treatment: a guide for physicians and other health professionals. New York (NY): Oxford University Press; 1998.
17. Asch A. Prenatal diagnosis and selective abortion: a challenge to practice and policy. Am J Public Health 1999;89:1649–57.
18. Parens E, Asch A. The disability rights critique of prenatal genetic testing. Reflections and Recommendations. Hastings Cent Rep 1999;29(5):S1–S22.
19. American College of Obstetricians and Gynecologists. Human resources. In: Guidelines for women's health care. 2nd ed. Washington, DC: ACOG; 2002. p. 13–31.

Informed Consent

Informed consent is an ethical concept that has become integral to contemporary medical ethics and medical practice. In recognition of the ethical importance of informed consent, the Committee on Ethics of the American College of Obstetricians and Gynecologists (ACOG) affirms the following 8 statements:

1. Informed consent for medical treatment, for participation in medical research, and for participation in teaching exercises involving students and residents is an ethical requirement that is partially reflected in legal doctrines and requirements.

2. Requiring informed consent is an expression of respect for the patient as a person; it particularly respects a patient's moral right to bodily integrity, to self-determination regarding sexuality and reproductive capacities, and to the support of the patient's freedom within caring relationships.

3. Informed consent not only ensures the protection of the patient against unwanted medical treatment, but it also makes possible the active involvement of the patient in her medical planning and care.

4. Communication is necessary if informed consent is to be realized, and physicians can help to find ways to facilitate communication not only in individual relations with patients but also in the structured context of medical care institutions.

5. Informed consent should be looked on as a process rather than a signature on a form. This process includes ongoing shared information

and developing choices as long as one is seeking medical assistance.

6. The ethical requirement of informed consent need not conflict with physicians' overall ethical obligation to a principle of beneficence; that is, every effort should be made to incorporate a commitment to informed consent within a commitment to provide medical benefit to patients and thus to respect them as whole and embodied persons.

7. When informed consent by the patient is impossible, a surrogate decision maker should be identified to represent the patient's wishes or best interests. In emergency situations, medical professionals may have to act according to their perceptions of the best interests of the patient; in rare instances, they may have to forgo obtaining consent because of some other overriding ethical obligation, such as protecting the public health.

8. Because ethical requirements and legal requirements cannot be equated, physicians also should acquaint themselves with federal and state legal requirements for informed consent.

The application of informed consent to contexts of obstetric and gynecologic practice invites ongoing clarification of the meaning of these 8 statements. What follows is an effort to provide this.

Historical Background

In 1980, the Committee on Ethics developed a statement on informed consent. This statement, "Ethical Considerations Associated with Informed Consent," was subsequently approved and issued in 1980 as a Statement of Policy by ACOG's Executive Board. In 1989, it was withdrawn for revision by the Committee on Ethics. The 1980 statement reflected what is now generally recognized as a paradigm shift

Previously published as Committee Opinion 108, May 1992; content revised January 2004 in the ethical understanding of the physician–patient relationship. The 1970s had seen in the United States a marked change from a traditional almost singular focus on the benefit of the patient as the governing ethical principle of medical care to a new and dramatic emphasis on a requirement of informed consent. That is, a central and often sole concern for the medical well-being of the patient gave way to, or was at least modified to include, concern for the patient's autonomy in making medical decisions.

In the 1980s this national shift was both reinforced and challenged in medical ethics. Clinical experience as well as developments in ethical theory generated further questions about the practice of informed consent and the legal doctrine that promoted it. If in the 1970s informed consent was embraced as a corrective to paternalism, the 1980s and 1990s exhibited a growing sense of the need for shared decision making as a corrective to the exaggerated individualism that patient autonomy had sometimes produced. At the same time, factors such as the proliferation of medical technologies, the bureaucratic and financial complexities of health care delivery systems, and the growing sophistication of the general public regarding medical limitations and possibilities continued to undergird an appreciation of the importance of patient autonomy and a demand for its safeguard in and through informed consent.

In the early 21st century, there are good reasons for considering once again the ethical significance and practical application of the requirement of informed consent. This is particularly true in the context of obstetric and gynecologic practice because medical options, public health problems, legal interventions, and political agendas have expanded and interconnected with one another in unprecedented ways. The concern of ACOG for these matters is reflected in its more recent documents on informed consent and on particular ethical problems such as maternal–fetal conflict, sterilization, and surgical options (see "Ethical Decision Making in Obstetrics and Gynecology" in Part I and "Patient Choice in the Maternal–Fetal Relationship," "Sterilization of Women, Including Those with Mental Disabilities," "Human Immunodeficiency Virus," and "Surgery and Patient Choice" in Part II) (1, 2). Although a general ethical doctrine of informed consent cannot by itself resolve problems like these, it is nonetheless necessary for understanding them.

Informed consent for medical treatment and for participation in medical research is both a legal and an ethical matter. In the recent history of informed consent, statutes and regulations as well as court decisions have played an important role in the identification and sanctioning of basic duties. Judicial decisions have sometimes provided insights regarding rights of self-determination and of privacy in the medical context. Government regulations have rendered operational some of the most general norms formulated in historic ethical codes*. Yet, there is little recent development in the legal doctrine of informed consent, and the most serious current questions are ethical ones before they become issues in the law. As the President's Commission reported in 1982, "Although the informed consent doctrine has substantial foundations in law, it is essentially an ethical imperative" (3). What above all bears reviewing, then, is the ethical dimension of the meaning, basis, and application of informed consent.

The Ethical Meaning of Informed Consent

The ethical concept of "informed consent" contains 2 major elements: 1) comprehension (or understanding) and 2) free consent. Both of these elements together constitute an important part of a patient's "self-determination" (the taking hold of her own life and action, determining the meaning and the possibility of what she undergoes as well as what she does).

Comprehension (as an ethical element in informed consent) includes awareness and understanding about the patient's situation and possibilities. It implies that she has been given adequate information about her diagnosis, prognosis, and alternative treatment choices, including the option of no treatment. Moreover, this information should be provided in language that is understandable to the particular patient, who may have linguistic or cognitive limitations. Comprehension in this sense is necessary for there to be freedom in consenting.

Free consent is an intentional and voluntary act that authorizes someone else to act in certain ways. In the context of medicine, it is an act by which an individual freely authorizes a medical intervention in

---

*The Nuremberg Code in 1948 and the World Medical Association's Declaration of Helsinki in 1964 identified ethical restrictions for medical research on human subjects. For a history of the development of such codes and a general history of the ethical and legal concept of informed consent, see Faden RR, Beauchamp TL. A history and theory of informed consent. New York (NY): Oxford University Press; 1986.

her life, whether in the form of treatment or participation in research. Consenting freely is incompatible with being coerced or unwillingly pressured by forces beyond herself. It involves the ability to choose among options and to choose other than what may be recommended.

Free consent, of course, admits of degrees, and its presence is not always verifiable in concrete instances. If it is to be operative at all in the course of medical treatment, it presupposes knowledge about and understanding of all the available options.

Many individuals who are thoughtful about these matters have different beliefs about the actual achievement of informed consent and about human freedom. Whether and what freedom itself is often has been disputed. These differences in underlying philosophical perspectives do not, however, alter the general agreement about the need for informed consent and about its basic ethical significance in the context of medical practice and research. It is still important to try to clarify, however, who and what informed consent serves, and how it may be protected and fostered. This clarification cannot be achieved without some continuing consideration of its basis and goals and the concrete contexts in which it must be realized.

The Ethical Basis and Purpose of Informed Consent

One of the important arguments for the ethical requirement of informed consent is an argument from utility, or from the benefit that can come to patients when they actively participate in decisions about their own medical care. That is, the involvement of patients in such decisions is good for their health—not only because it helps protect against treatment that patients might consider harmful, but because it contributes positively to their well-being. There are at least 2 presuppositions here: 1) patients know something experientially about their own medical condition that can be helpful and even necessary to the sound management of their medical care and 2) wherever it is possible, the active role of primary guardian of their own health is more conducive to well-being than is a passive and submissive "sick role." The positive benefits of patient decision making are obvious, for example, in the treatment of alcohol abuse. But the benefits of active participation in medical decisions are multifold for patients, whether they are trying to maintain their general health, recover from illness, conceive and give birth to healthy newborns, live responsible sexual lives, or accept the limits of medical technology.

Utility, however, is not the only reason for protecting and promoting patient decision making. Indeed, the most commonly accepted foundation for informed consent is the principle of respect for persons. This principle expresses an ethical requirement to treat persons as "ends in themselves" (that is, not to use them solely as means or instruments for someone else's purposes and goals). The logic of this requirement is based on the perception that all persons, as persons, have certain features or characteristics that constitute the source of an inherent dignity, a worthiness and claim to be affirmed in their own right. One of these features has come to be identified as autonomy—a person's capacity or at least potential for self-determination (for self-governance and freedom of choice). To be autonomous is to have the capacity to set one's own agenda. Given this capacity in persons, it is ordinarily an ethically unacceptable violation of who and what persons are to coerce their actions or to refuse their participation in important decisions that affect their lives.

One of the important developments in ethical theory in recent years is the widespread recognition that autonomy is not the only characteristic of persons that is a basis for the requirement of respect. Human beings are essentially social beings, relational in the structure of their personalities, their needs, and their possibilities. Given this "relationality," then, the goal of human life and the content of human well-being cannot be adequately understood only in terms of self-determination—especially if self-determination is understood individualistically and if it results in human relationships that are primarily adversarial. A sole or even central emphasis on patient autonomy in the informed consent process in the medical context risks replacing paternalism with a distanced and impersonal relationship of strangers negotiating rights and duties. If persons are to be respected and their well-being promoted, informed consent must be seen as expressing a fuller notion of relationship.

Patients come to medical decisions with a history of relationships, personal and social, familial and institutional. Decisions are made in the context of these relationships, shared or not shared, as the situation allows. Specifically, these decisions are made in a relationship between patient and physician (or often between patient and multiple professional caregivers).

The focus, then, for understanding both the basis and the content of informed consent must shift to include the many facets of the physician–patient relationship. Informed consent, from this point of view, is not an end, but a means. It is a means not only to the responsible participation by patients in their own medical care; it also is a means to a new form of relationship between physician (or any medical caregiver) and patient. From this perspective, it is possible to see the contradictions inherent in an approach to informed consent that would, for example:

- Lead a physician (or anyone else) to say of a patient, "I gave her informed consent"
- Assume that informed consent was achieved simply by the signing of a document
- Consider informed consent primarily as a safeguard for physicians against medical liability

It also is possible to see, from this perspective, that informed consent is not meant to undergird a patient's unlimited demand for treatment or choice of treatment modalities that are medically inadvisable. Respecting the patient's autonomy means that the physician cannot impose treatments; it does not mean that the physician must provide treatment, especially if the physician considers it inappropriate or harmful.

Obstetrics and Gynecology: Special Ethical Concerns for Informed Consent

The practice of obstetrics and gynecology has always faced special ethical questions in the implementation of informed consent. How, for example, can the autonomy of patients best be respected when serious decisions must be made in the challenging situations of labor and delivery? What kinds of guidelines can physicians find for respecting the autonomy of adolescents, when society acknowledges this autonomy by and large only in the limited spheres of sexuality and reproduction? In the context of genetic counseling, where being "nondirective" is the norm, is it ever appropriate to recommend a specific course of action? How much information should be given to patients about controversies surrounding specific treatments? How are beneficence requirements (regarding the well-being of the patient) to be balanced with the rights of patient choice, especially in a field of medical practice where so many key decisions are irreversible? These and many other questions continue to be important for fulfilling the ethical requirement of informed consent.

Developments in the ethical doctrine of informed consent (regarding, for example, the significance that relationships have for decision making) have helped to focus some of the concerns that are particular to the practice of obstetrics and gynecology. Where women's health care needs are addressed, and especially where these needs are related to women's sexuality and reproductive capacities, the issues of patient autonomy and relationality take on special significance. In other words, the gender of patients makes a difference where ethical questions of informed consent are concerned, because gender in our society has been a relevant factor in interpreting the meaning of autonomy and relationality. This is not to say that in some essential sense autonomy or relationality (or informed consent and relationships) ought to be different for women and men; indeed, quite the opposite. The ethical requirement of informed consent in its essential elements applies equally to men and women.

Although issues of gender are to be found in every area of medical practice and research[†], they are particularly important in the area of obstetrics and gynecology. Of special relevance here, for example, are the insights now being articulated by women out of their experience—that is, their experience specifically in the medical setting, but also more generally in relation to their own bodies, in various patterns of relation with other individuals, and in the larger societal and institutional contexts in which they live. These insights offer both a help and an ongoing challenge to the professional self-understanding and practice of obstetricians and gynecologists (whether they themselves are women or men).

Obstetrics and gynecology has in a special way seen new dimensions of informed consent emerge, and here new models for the active participation of health care recipients have been created. Some of these developments are the result of effective arguments that pregnancy and childbirth are not diseases, although they bring women importantly into relation with medical professionals. Even when women's medical needs are more precisely needs for diagno-

---

[†]See, for example, a study of court decisions on refusal of treatment regarding dying patients (Miles SH, August A. Courts, gender, and "the right to die." Law Med Health Care 1990;18:85–95). The conclusion of this study is that court decisions for women patients differ from court decisions for men; that is, generally, men's previously stated wishes about "extraordinary" or "heroic" measures of treatment are taken more seriously than are women's.

sis and treatment, their concerns to hold together the values of both autonomy and relationality have been influential in shaping not only ethical theory but also medical practice. Women themselves have questioned, for example, whether autonomy can really be protected if it is addressed in a vacuum, apart from an individual's concrete roles and relationships. But women as well as men also have recognized the ongoing importance of respect for autonomy as a requirement of moral justice in every relationship. Many women therefore continue to articulate fundamental concerns for bodily integrity and self-determination. At the same time, they call for attention to the complexity of the relationships that are involved when sexuality and parenting are at issue in medical care.

The difficulties that beset the full achievement of informed consent in the practice of obstetrics and gynecology are not limited to individual and interpersonal factors. Both providers and recipients of medical care within this specialty have recognized the influence of such broad social problems as the historical imbalance of power in gender relations, the constraints on individual choice posed by complex medical technology, and the intersection of gender bias with race and class bias in the attitudes and actions of individuals and institutions. None of these problems makes the achievement of informed consent impossible. But, they alert us to the need to identify the conditions and limits, as well as the central requirements, of the ethical application of this doctrine.

Ethical Applications of Informed Consent

Insofar as comprehension and free consent are the basic ethical elements in informed consent, its efficacy and adequacy will depend on the fullness of their realization in patients' decisions. There are ways of assessing this and strategies for achieving it, even though—like every event of human freedom—informed consent involves a process that is not subject to precise measurement.

It is difficult to specify what consent consists of and requires, because it is difficult to describe a free decision in the abstract. Two things can be said about it in the context of informed consent to a medical intervention, however, elaborating on the conceptual elements we have already identified. The first is to describe what consent is not, what it is freedom from. Informed consent includes freedom from external coercion, manipulation, or infringe-

ment of bodily integrity. It is freedom from being acted on by others when they have not taken account of and respected the individual's own preference and choice. This kind of freedom for a patient is not incompatible with a physician's giving reasons that favor one option over another. Medical recommendations, when they are not coercive or deceptive, do not violate the requirements of informed consent. For example, to try to convince a patient to take a medication that will improve her health is not to take away her freedom (assuming that the methods of convincing are ones that respect and address, not overwhelm, her freedom).

The second thing that can be said about informed consent to a medical intervention is that although it may be an authorization of someone else's action toward one's self, it is—more profoundly—an active participation in decisions about the management of one's medical care. It is therefore (or can be) not only a "permitting" but a "doing." It can include decisions to make every effort toward a cure of a disease; or when cure is no longer a reasonable goal, to maintain functional equilibrium; or, finally, to receive medical care primarily in the form of comfort only. The variety of choices that are possible to a patient ranges, for example, from surgery to medical therapy, from diagnostic tests to menopausal hormone therapy, and from one form of contraception to another. For women in the context of obstetrics and gynecology, the choices often are ones of positive determination of one kind of assisted reproduction or another or one kind of preventive medicine or another—choices that are best described as determinations of their own actions rather than the "receiving" of care as a "patient."

Consent in this sense requires not only external freedom and freedom from inner compulsion, but also (as we have already observed) freedom from ignorance. Hence, consent is required to be "informed."

Consent is based on the disclosure of information and a sharing of interpretations of its meaning by a medical professional. The accuracy of disclosure, insofar as it is possible, is governed by the ethical requirement of truth-telling. The adequacy of disclosure has been judged by various criteria, which may include:

1. The common practice of the profession
2. The reasonable needs and expectations of the ordinary individual who might be making a particular decision

3. The unique needs of an individual patient faced with a given choice‡

Although these criteria have been generated in the rulings of courts, the courts themselves have not provided a unified voice as to which of these criteria should be determinative. Trends in judicial decisions in most states were for a time primarily in the direction of the "professional practice" criterion, requiring only the consistency of a physician's disclosure with the practice of disclosure by other physicians. Now the trend in many states is more clearly toward the "reasonable person" criterion, holding the medical profession to the standard of what is judged to be material to an ordinary individual's decision in the given medical situation. The criterion of the subjective needs of the patient in question generally has been too difficult to implement in the legal arena, although the force of its ethical appeal is significant.

Health care providers should engage in some ethical discernment of their own as to which criteria are most faithful to the needs and rightful claims of patients for disclosure. All 3 criteria offer reminders of ethical accountability and guidelines for practice. All 3 can help to illuminate what needs to be shared in the significant categories for disclosure: diagnosis and description of the patient's medical condition, description of the proposed treatment and its nature and purpose, risks and possible complications associated with the treatment, alternative treatments or the relative merits of no treatment at all, and the probability of success of the treatment.

Listing categories of disclosure does not by itself include all the elements that are important to adequacy of disclosure. For example, the obligation to provide adequate information to a patient implies an obligation for physicians to be current in their own knowledge, for example, about treatments and disease processes. As an aid to physicians in communicating information to patients, ACOG makes available more than 100 patient education pamphlets on a wide variety of subjects. The pamphlet on cystic fibrosis carrier testing is explicitly intended to provide information essential to an informed choice; it includes a form for consenting to or declining carrier testing (4). When physicians make informed consent possible for patients by giving them the knowledge they need for choice, it should be clear to patients that their continued medical care by a given

physician is not contingent on their making the choice that the physician prefers (assuming the limited justifiable exceptions to this that will be addressed later).

Those who are most concerned with problems of informed consent insist that central to its achievement is communication—communication between physician and patient, communication among the many medical professionals who are involved in the care of the patient, and communication (where this is possible and appropriate) with the family of the patient. The role of documentation in a formal process of informed consent can be a help to necessary communication (depending on the methods and manner of its implementation). The completion of consent forms, however legally significant, cannot substitute for the communication of disclosure, the conversation that leads to free refusal or consent (1, 5).

To focus on the importance of communication for the implementation of an ethical doctrine of informed consent is, then, to underline the fact that informed consent involves a process. There is a process of communication that leads to initial consent (or refusal to consent) and that can make possible appropriate ongoing decision making.

There are, of course, practical difficulties with ensuring the kind of communication necessary for informed consent. Limitations of time in a clinical context, patterns of authority uncritically maintained, underdeveloped professional communication skills, "language barriers" between technical discourse and ordinarily comprehensible expression, and situations of stress on all sides—all of these frequently yield less than ideal circumstances for communication. Yet the ethical requirement of informed consent, no less than a requirement for good medical care, extends to a requirement for reasonable communication. The conditions for communication may be enhanced by creating institutional policies and structures that make it more possible and effective.

It is obvious that although disclosure and consent are basic ethical requirements and not only ideals, they admit of degrees. There will always be varying levels of understanding, varying degrees of internal freedom. The very matters of disclosure are of a kind that often are characterized by disagreement among professionals, uncertainty and fallibility in everyone's judgments, the results not only of scientific analysis but of medical insight and art. And the capacities of patients for comprehension and consent are more or less acute, of greater or lesser power, focused in weak or strong personal

---

‡For an overview of legal standards for disclosure and ethical questions that go beyond legal standards, see Faden RR, Beauchamp TL. A history and theory of informed consent. New York (NY): Oxford University Press; 1986.

integration, and compromised or not by pain, medication, or disease. Some limitations mitigate the obligation of informed consent, and some render it impossible. But any compromise or relaxation of the full ethical obligation of informed consent requires specific ethical justification.

The Limits of Informed Consent

Because informed consent admits of degrees of implementation, there are limits to its achievement. These are not only the limits of fallible knowledge or imperfect communication. They are limitations in the capacity of patients for comprehension and for choice. Assessment of patient capacity is itself a complex matter, subject to mistakes and to bias. Hence, a great deal of attention has been given to criteria for determining individual capacity (and the legally defined characteristic of "competence") and for just procedures for its evaluation (3). When individuals are entirely incapacitated for informed consent, the principle of respect for persons requires that they be protected. In these situations, someone else must make decisions on behalf of the patient. A surrogate decision maker should be identified to provide a "substituted judgment" (a decision based on what the patient would have wanted, assuming some knowledge of what the patient's wishes would be); if the patient's wishes are unknown, the surrogate makes a decision according to the "best interests" of the patient. If the patient has previously executed an advance directive, that document should guide the selection of a surrogate decision maker as well as the specific decisions made by the surrogate.

The judgment that informed consent is impossible in some circumstances indicates a kind of limit that is different from a partial actualization of consent or a consent by an appropriate surrogate. One way to acknowledge this is to say that there are limits to the obligation to obtain informed consent at all. There are several exceptions to the strict rule of informed consent.

First, impossibility of any achievement of informed consent suspends or limits the ethical obligation. This is exemplified in emergency situations in which consent is unattainable and in other situations when a patient is not at all competent or capable of giving consent and an appropriate surrogate decision maker is not available. In the practice of obstetrics and gynecology, as in any other specialty practice, there are situations where decisions can be based only on what is judged to be in the best interest of the patient—a judgment made, if possible, by

a designated surrogate, legal guardian, or family members together with medical professionals. Yet often when a patient is not able to decide for herself (perhaps, for example, because of the amount of medication needed to control pain), a substituted judgment or a judgment on the basis of prior informed consent can be made with confidence if care has been taken beforehand to learn the patient's wishes. This signals the importance of early communication so that what a patient would choose in a developing situation is known—so that, indeed, it remains possible to respect the self-determination that informed consent represents.

A second way in which the rule of informed consent may be suspended or limited is by being overridden by another obligation. There are a number of other ethical obligations that can, in certain circumstances, override or set limits to the extent of the requirement of informed consent. For example, strong claims for the public good (specifically, public health) may set limits to what a patient can choose or refuse. That is, the rights of others not to be harmed may sometimes take priority over an individual's right to refuse a medical procedure (as is the case in exceptional forms of mandatory medical testing and reporting). On the other hand, scarcity of personnel and equipment may in some circumstances mean that individual patients cannot have certain medical procedures "just for the choosing."

In rare circumstances, what is known as therapeutic privilege can override an obligation to disclose information and hence to obtain informed consent. Therapeutic privilege is the limited privilege of a physician to withhold information from a patient in the belief that this information about the patient's medical condition and options will seriously harm the patient. Concern for the patient's well-being (the obligation of beneficence) thus comes into conflict with respect for the patient's autonomy. This is a difficult notion to apply—great caution must be taken in any appeal made to it—and the rationale for withholding information should be carefully documented. The concept of therapeutic privilege should not, for example, be used as a justification for ignoring the needs and rights of adolescents to participate in decisions about their sexuality and their reproductive capacities. It is reasonable to argue that therapeutic privilege is almost never a basis for permanently overriding the obligation of informed consent. Ordinarily such overriding represents a temporary situation, one that will later allow the kind of communication conducive to the restored freedom of the patient.

Sometimes another exception to the rule of informed consent is thought to occur in the rare situation when a patient effectively *waives* her right to give it. This can take the form of refusing information necessary for an informed decision, or simply refusing altogether to make any decision. However, the following 2 statements are reasons for not considering this an exception of the same type as the other exceptions:

1. A waiver in such instances seems to be itself an exercise of choice, and its acceptance can be part of respect for the patient's autonomy.
2. Implicit in the ethical concept of informed consent is the goal of maximizing a patient's freedoms, which means that waivers should not be accepted complacently without some concern for the causes of the patient's desire not to participate in the management of her care.

In any case, it should be noted that in states where written documentation of informed consent is required, it may be necessary to meet this requirement in some legally acceptable way.

Finally, there are limits intrinsic to the patient–physician relationship that keep the requirement of informed consent from ever being absolute. Physicians also are moral agents or decision makers, and, as such, retain areas of free choice—as in the freedom not to provide medical care that they deem medically or ethically irresponsible (a freedom that is sometimes called a right to "conscientious objection"). Interpretations of medical need and usefulness may lead a physician, for example, to refuse to perform surgery or prescribe medication (although the physician should provide the patient with information about her medical options). In the mutuality of the patient–physician relationship, each one is to be respected as a person and supported in her or his autonomous decisions insofar as those decisions are not, in particular circumstances, overridden by other ethical obligations. The existing imbalance of power in this relationship, however, is a reminder to physicians of their greater obligation to ensure and facilitate the informed consent of each patient. That is, differences in professional knowledge can and should be bridged precisely through efforts at communication of information. Only in this way can decisions that are truly mutual be achieved.

Acknowledging the limits of the ethical requirement of informed consent, then, clarifies but does not weaken the requirement as such. In recognition of this, the Committee on Ethics affirms the 8 statements that were presented at the beginning of this chapter.

References

1. American College of Obstetricians and Gynecologists. The assistant: information for improved risk management. Washington, DC: ACOG; 2001.
2. American College of Obstetricians and Gynecologists. Professional liability and risk management: a resource for obstetrician–gynecologists in training and in practice. Washington, DC: ACOG; 2002.
3. President's Commission for the Study of Ethical Problems in Medicine and Biomedical and Behavioral Research. Making health care decisions: the ethical and legal implications of informed consent in the patient-practitioner relationship. Vol 1. Washington, DC: U.S. Government Printing Office; 1982.
4. American College of Obstetricians and Gynecologists. Cystic fibrosis carrier testing: the decision is yours. ACOG Patient Education Pamphlet CF001. Washington, DC: ACOG; 2001.
5. American Medical Association. Medicolegal forms with legal analysis. Chicago (IL): AMA; 1999.

Bibliography

Beauchamp TL, Childress JF. Principles of biomedical ethics. 5th ed. New York (NY): Oxford University Press; 2001.

Berg JW, Appelbaum PS, Lidz CW, Parker LS. Informed consent: legal theory and clinical practice. New York (NY): Oxford University Press; 2001.

Faden RR, Beauchamp TL. A history and theory of informed consent. New York (NY): Oxford University Press; 1986.

Katz J. The silent world of doctor and patient. New York (NY): The Free Press; 1984.

Levine RJ. Ethics and regulation of clinical research. 2nd ed. New Haven (CT): Yale University Press; 1988.

President's Commission for the Study of Ethical Problems in Medicine and Biomedical and Behavioral Research. Making health care decisions: the ethical and legal implications of informed consent in the patient-practitioner relationship. Vol 1. Washington, DC: U.S. Government Printing Office; 1982.

President's Commission for the Study of Ethical Problems in Medicine and Biomedical and Behavioral Research. Making health care decisions: the ethical and legal implications of informed consent in the patient-practitioner relationship. Vol 2. Washington, DC: U.S. Government Printing Office; 1982.

President's Commission for the Study of Ethical Problems in Medicine and Biomedical and Behavioral Research. Making health care decisions: the ethical and legal implications of informed consent in the patient-practitioner relationship. Vol 3. Washington, DC: U.S. Government Printing Office; 1982.

Suggested Reading

Braddock CH 3rd, Edwards KA, Hasenberg NM, Laidley TL, Levinson W. Informed decision making in outpatient practice: time to get back to basics. JAMA 1999;282:2313–20.

Informed consent and the use of gametes and embryos for research. The Ethics Committee of the American Society for Reproductive Medicine. Fertil Steril 1997;68:780–1.

International Federation of Gynecology and Obstetrics (FIGO). Guidelines regarding informed consent. In: Recommendations on ethical issues in obstetrics and gynecology by the FIGO Committee for the Ethical Aspects of Human Reproduction and Women's Health. London: FIGO; 2000. p. 10–1.

National Bioethics Advisory Commission. Ethical and policy issues in international research: clinical trials in developing countries. Vols 1–2. Bethesda (MD): NBAC; 2001.

National Bioethics Advisory Commission. Ethical and policy issues in research involving human participants. Vols 1–2. Bethesda (MD): NBAC; 2001.

PART II
Caring for Patients

"The patient–physician relationship is the central focus of all ethical concerns, and the welfare of the patient should form the basis of all medical judgments"—"Code of Professional Ethics of the American College of Obstetricians and Gynecologists"

For most obstetrician–gynecologists, the core of their professional duties is caring for patients. In its Practice Bulletins, Committee Opinions, guidelines books, and other documents, the American College of Obstetricians and Gynecologists offers clinical practice guidelines to assist clinicians in making medical judgments. But ensuring the welfare of the patient is not a matter of simply understanding what procedures are medically indicated and being able to perform them proficiently. It also depends on the ability of the clinician to apply ethical principles to the provision of specific health care services.

The aim of this part of Ethics in Obstetrics and Gynecology *is to assist obstetrician–gynecologists in conducting a useful ethical analysis for a range of medical and surgical procedures commonly performed in women. It begins with a process for guiding obstetrician–gynecologists in making ethical decisions about surgical procedures, and it illustrates this process with chapters on specific procedures spanning from the beginning to the end of life and addressing the unique maternal–fetal relationship.*

Surgery and Patient Choice

Is it ethical to perform an elective cesarean delivery for a woman with a normal pregnancy, a prophylactic oophorectomy for a 30-year-old patient with no family history of ovarian cancer, or a tubal ligation for an 18-year-old nulligravid woman? How should the physician respond to a patient who requests a specific surgical therapy without having an accepted medical indication? Should health care options be regarded in the same way as choice of cereal in the supermarket: the consumer makes a choice based on appearance, content, and cost, and the grocer takes the money and bags the cornflakes, without providing any direction? Is choosing a medical procedure so radically different and complex that this analogy is inappropriate?

Years ago, patients presented to their physicians with symptoms, and the physicians would establish diagnoses then make recommendations for therapy; usually recommendations were accepted by patients without question. An example of that paternalistic model was the widespread practice of "twilight sleep" for labor and delivery. Physicians administered a narcotic and scopolamine, and decisions during labor and delivery were delegated to the medical team. In contrast, today the first prenatal visit may open with a discussion of the patient's birth plan, including her preferences for anesthesia, episiotomy, forceps use, cesarean delivery, and breastfeeding. The purpose of this chapter is to provide the obstetrician–gynecologist with an approach to decision making based on ethics in an environment of increased patient information, recognition of patient autonomy, direct-to-consumer marketing, and a plethora of alternative, investigational, or unproven treatments for many conditions.

Previously published as Committee Opinion 289, November 2003

Ethical Principles

Decision making in obstetrics and gynecology should be guided by the ethical principles of respect for patient autonomy, beneficence, nonmaleficence, justice, and veracity and as set forth throughout this document and in the "Code of Professional Ethics of the American College of Obstetricians and Gynecologists" (see Appendix). In addition, the obstetrician–gynecologist must consider resolution of conflicts of interest, acknowledgment of the profession's responsibility to society as a whole, and the maintenance of the dignity and honor of the discipline of obstetrics and gynecology and its standards of care. This chapter will address issues related to surgery; however, the ethical principles are the same as for other health care decisions (eg, diagnostic testing or medical therapy).

Patient autonomy and the concept of informed consent or refusal are central to issues regarding patient choice to have or not have a surgical procedure. It is the obligation of the obstetrician–gynecologist to fully inform the patient regarding treatment options and the potential risks and benefits of those options. In discussing these options, the physician should take into account the context of the patient's decision making, including the potential influences of family and society (1). Once the physician is satisfied that the patient fully comprehends the options, her autonomous decision ordinarily should be respected and supported. Patients should be encouraged to seek second opinions when in doubt or in need of reassurance. However, even though the decision of the patient should be respected, this might not include supporting the decision, particularly when doing so is in direct conflict with other guiding ethical principles. At times, these other principles may take priority over supporting the patient's decisions.

The principle of *beneficence* refers to the ethical obligation of the physician to promote the health and welfare of the patient. The complementary principle of *nonmaleficence* refers to the physician's obligation to not harm the patient. When a patient refuses a surgery or other treatment that the obstetrician–gynecologist believes is necessary for her health and welfare, beneficence and nonmaleficence can conflict with patient *autonomy*. In almost all situations, the patient has a right to refuse unwanted treatment. She does not, however, have a parallel right to demand treatment that the physician believes is unwise or overly risky.

Justice, as an ethical principle, applies to the physician, the hospital, the payer, and society, as well as to the individual patient. Although there are many theories of justice, in the medical context this principle requires that medical professionals treat individuals fairly. It is important for the physician to consider the impact on not only the individual patient, but also society. At the level of the physician–patient relationship, justice implies, for instance, that physicians consider a patient's request for an elective procedure in the context of similar types of requests by other patients. At the societal level, justice directs physicians to consider the impact of their decision to perform a procedure in terms of the allocation of scarce resources.

The ethical principle of *veracity*, or truth telling, is important in surgical counseling and decision making. When the patient requests a procedure to which the physician is morally opposed (such as abortion or permanent sterilization), it is the right of the physician to refuse to provide the service. However, the physician must convey to the patient that this refusal is based on moral, not medical, grounds. The obstetrician–gynecologist should not misrepresent his or her experience with the proposed treatment or knowledge regarding potential long-term outcomes.

The Physician–Patient Relationship

The relationship between the physician and patient can take 4 forms (2). Depending on which model is used, different ethical principles emerge as relevant to ethical decision making. The ideal model for the physician–patient relationship has been the subject of considerable debate. In fact, physicians probably use all 4 models, depending on the individual patient and disease process involved (2).

Paternalistic Model

In the paternalistic physician–patient model (2), the physician might present only information on risks and benefits of a procedure that he or she thinks will lead the patient to making the "right" (ie, in this model, the physician-supported) decision regarding care. One example of the paternalistic model would be recommending amniocentesis for a 35-year-old pregnant patient but offering no alternatives.

This model is not appropriate when the patient is competent to make informed decisions, but it may be the best choice in situations of last resort, such as unconscious patients in the emergency department when no family member is present. When the patient is ill and unable to engage, either physically or mentally, in a discussion of the risks and benefits of a particular surgical intervention and there is neither an advance directive nor an assigned proxy for health care decisions, a paternalistic physician–patient relationship may be the best way to balance the ethical principles of beneficence and nonmaleficence with impaired patient autonomy.

Informative Model

At the opposite end of the spectrum, the informative model describes a physician–patient relationship in which the physician is a provider of objective and technical information regarding the patient's medical problem and its potential therapeutic solutions. The patient has complete control over surgical decision making, and the physician's values are not discussed. An example is a physician offering a patient with an abnormal cervical cytology the options of colposcopy, loop electrosurgical excision procedure, laser ablation, cold knife conization, and hysterectomy. The discussion includes a complete description of advantages, disadvantages, risks, and complications of each option. The discussion does not include any statement about the physician's recommendations or prioritization of the options.

A serious drawback of this model is the physician's abandonment of the role of a caring partner and medical expert in the decision-making process. This model also assumes that patients have set values and are able to completely integrate the sometimes-complex medical and surgical treatment decisions with those values. However, when the physician–patient relationship is necessarily brief and there are multiple treatment options with roughly equal risks and benefits, the informative model may be appropriate. One example is the choice of having a genetic amniocentesis for advanced maternal age versus multiple marker testing or no testing.

One of the many unfortunate consequences of the professional liability crisis is the unsubstantiated belief of some physicians that the informative model reduces the physician's risk of liability. Such a belief raises concerns about physicians protecting themselves rather than working in the best interests of their patients.

This model may not be ideal for patient care in most situations because the physician's professional judgment is generally of considerable value to patients. In any case, it probably is impossible for a physician to counsel a patient with complete objectivity and without introducing some implied preference for one of many options (3).

Interpretive Model

Other models for physician–patient relationships strike a middle ground between the extremes of the paternalistic and informative models. In the interpretive model, the physician helps the patient clarify and integrate her values into the decision-making process, while acting as an information source regarding the technical aspects of any given medical procedure. In this model the physician aids the patient in "self-understanding; the patient comes to know more clearly who he or she is and how various medical options bear on his or her identity" (2).

Application of this model to an example of cervical dysplasia might result in the physician noting that the patient was bothered by menses, had completed her childbearing, and was very fearful of cancer. On that basis the physician recommends hysterectomy over other options. When implementing this model, the physician must be careful to help the patient clarify her values while not imposing his or her own values or beliefs.

Deliberative Model

In the deliberative model, the physician's role is to guide the patient in taking the most admirable or moral (based on her values, needs, and fears) course of treatment or health-related action (2). It is similar to the interpretive model in that it includes a discussion of not only the medical benefits and risks, but also the patient's individual priorities, values, and fears. It goes beyond the interpretive model in that the physician must consciously communicate to the patient his or her health values. However, the physician should not use the moral discussion to dictate to the patient the "best" course of action (2). Because of the potential for an unequal balance of power in the physician–patient relationship, care should be taken in this model to avoid subjecting the patient to undue pressure.

The Process of Decision Making

Each physician should exercise judgment when determining whether information presented to the patient is adequate. The practice of evidence-based medicine involves understanding the scientific basis of treatment and the strength of the evidence and applying the results of the strongest evidence available to medical decision making. Frequently, both surgical and medical decisions need to be made in a context in which the scientific evidence supporting one treatment option over another is incomplete, of poor quality, or totally lacking. There is no ethical imperative to initiate discussion of treatment options that are unproved, "innovative" (ie, performed somewhere without evidence of relative efficacy, risks, and the like), or complementary and alternative medicine without evidence. The physician may, however, want to discuss investigational options so that the patient understands the unproven nature of these options and can make an informed decision about them. Surgical and medical advice or guidance for many obstetric and gynecologic problems is based in part on science, in part on the experience and values of the physician, and in part on the physician's understanding of the patient's preferences, values, and desired outcome.

When working with a patient to make decisions about surgery, it is important for obstetricians and gynecologists to take a broad view of the consequences of surgical treatment and to acknowledge the lack of firm evidence for the benefit of one approach over another when no evidence exists. For example, a discussion of treatment options for menorrhagia associated with leiomyoma should include the fact that the long-term risks and benefits of the multiple treatment options have not been compared directly (4). Recommendation for a particular option is dictated by many factors, including patient age, leiomyoma size, bleeding severity, and coexisting medical conditions, but in many cases 2 or more therapeutic options probably would be regarded as equally medically sound. Comparing possible long-term complications of hysterectomy (such as bowel obstruction and loss of vaginal support) with the risks of more conservative surgical approaches (such as the possible need for future treatment of recurrent leiomyomata) is an important part of informed consent. Helping patients understand potential long- and short-term consequences of any given decision, as well as giving patients an appreciation of the quality of evidence on which each option is based, is a critical part of informed consent. In addition, the physician must be aware of potential personal conflicts of interest that may be present, such as personal financial gain related to the provision or non-provision of surgical care, and he or she must guard against this as an influence when giving guidance to patients as they make treatment choices.

Elective Cesarean Delivery: An Example of the Process

In obstetrics, the ethical issues of informed consent and patient choice are exemplified in the current debate regarding whether elective cesarean delivery should be offered as a birth option in normal pregnancy (5). The wide range of opinion on this issue is reflected in the language that is used, with varying terms reflecting different views of the physician–patient relationship. "Cesarean delivery on demand" reflects the informative model, in which the physician simply describes options and provides the service chosen by the patient. The phrase "elective cesarean delivery" is more suggestive of the deliberative and interpretive models, in which the physician and patient discuss concerns, needs, values, and the like.

The ethical evaluation is clouded by the limitations of data regarding relative short- and long-term risks and benefits of cesarean versus vaginal delivery. For example, limitations that need to be acknowledged on both sides of the debate include evidence for long-term reduction in pelvic floor disorders in women undergoing elective cesarean delivery and lack of extensive morbidity and mortality data comparing routine cesarean delivery with vaginal birth.

Each of the ethical principles contributes to the decision-making process regarding elective cesarean delivery. However, none alone is sufficient for making the decision.

If taken in a vacuum, the principle of patient autonomy would lend support to the permissibility of elective cesarean delivery in a normal pregnancy, after adequate informed consent. To ensure that the patient's consent is, in fact, informed, the physician should explore the patient's concerns. For example, a patient may request elective cesarean delivery because she is afraid of discomfort during labor (6). In this case, providing her with information about procedures available for effective pain relief during labor may result in an agreement to proceed without surgery (7).

The ethical principle of justice regarding the allocation of medical resources must be considered in the debate over elective cesarean delivery and informed patient choice. It is not clear whether widespread implementation of elective cesarean birth would increase or decrease resources required to provide delivery services. Comprehensive analysis of costs and benefits for current and subsequent pregnancies would provide a basis for application of the principle of justice (8).

The application of the principles of beneficence and nonmaleficence (a physician should offer only treatments that promote the health and welfare of the patient) is made problematic by the limitations of the scientific data described previously. Different interpretations of the risks and benefits are the basis for reasonable differences among obstetricians regarding this challenging issue. How certain are we that elective cesarean delivery really protects pelvic support 20 years later? How different is the maternal mortality of an elective or repeat cesarean delivery in a healthy woman compared with that of a woman who has had 1 or 2 vaginal deliveries? Are there any desirable or undesirable psychosocial effects of elective cesarean delivery? The currently available data do not adequately represent the comparative populations in question. For instance, data regarding outcomes of cesarean delivery usually involve complicated pregnancies or women in whom a trial of labor has failed. These outcomes are compared with those involving probably healthier women who were able to deliver vaginally. As better data accumulate, the principle of beneficence may result in a shift in clinical practice.

Based on these principles, is it ethical to agree to a patient request for elective cesarean birth in the absence of an accepted medical indication? The response must begin with the physician's assessment of the current data regarding the relative benefits and risks of the 2 approaches. In the absence of significant data on the risks and benefits of cesarean delivery, the burden of proof should fall on those who are advocates for a change in policy in support of elective cesarean delivery (ie, the replacement of a natural process with a major surgical procedure). If the physician believes that cesarean delivery promotes the overall health and welfare of the woman and her fetus more than vaginal birth, he or she is ethically justified in performing a cesarean delivery. Similarly, if the physician believes that performing a cesarean delivery would be detrimental to the overall health and welfare of the woman and her fetus, he or she is ethically obliged to refrain from performing the surgery. In this case, a referral to another health care provider would be appropriate if the physician and patient cannot agree on a route of delivery.

Finally, given the lack of data, it is not ethically necessary to initiate discussion regarding the relative risks and benefits of elective cesarean birth versus vaginal delivery with every pregnant patient. There is no obligation to initiate discussion about procedures that the physician does not consider medically acceptable or are unproved.

Using the ethical principles of beneficence and patient autonomy, an algorithm has been proposed for deciding between the performance of a cesarean delivery and making a referral in cases in which the physician's recommendation is vaginal delivery and the informed patient makes the autonomous decision to request a cesarean delivery (9). For a discussion of other special considerations involving patient choice in obstetric decision making, the reader is referred to "Patient Choice in the Maternal–Fetal Relationship" in Part II.

Summary

Although informed refusal of care by the patient is a familiar situation for most clinicians in both obstetrics and gynecology, acknowledgment of the importance of patient autonomy and increased patient access to information (such as on the Internet) has prompted more patient-generated requests for surgical interventions not necessarily recommended by their physicians. A patient request for elective cesarean delivery, prompted by a perception of lower risk to the woman (of pelvic floor and sexual dysfunction) and fetus with cesarean birth, is an obstetric example. Other examples include requests for prophylactic oophorectomy to reduce risk of ovarian cancer in otherwise healthy, low-risk women.

The response to such requests must begin with the physician having a good understanding of the scientific evidence for and against the requested procedure. With that information, the physician should counsel the patient within the framework of the ethical principles of autonomy, beneficence, nonmaleficence, veracity, and justice. The ethical models described in this document provide an approach for using these principles. The physician should use the opportunity that this kind of request presents to explore the patient's concerns. In most cases, providing information and careful counseling will allow patients and their physicians to reach a mutually acceptable decision. If an acceptable balance cannot be reached by the patient and physician, the patient may choose to continue care with another provider.

References

1. Mackenzie C, Stoljar N, editors. Relational autonomy: feminist perspectives on autonomy, agency, and the social self. New York (NY): Oxford University Press; 2000.
2. Emanuel EJ, Emanuel LL. Four models of the physician-patient relationship. JAMA 1992;267:2221–6.
3. Mahowald MB. On the treatment of myopia: feminist standpoint theory and bioethics. In: Wolf S, editor. Feminism and bioethics: beyond reproduction. New York (NY): Oxford University Press; 1996. p. 95–115.
4. Myers ER, Barber MD, Gustilo-Ashby T, Couchman G, Matchar DB, McCrory DC. Management of uterine leiomyomata: what do we really know? Obstet Gynecol 2002;100:8–17.
5. Minkoff H, Chervenak FA. Elective primary cesarean delivery. N Engl J Med 2003;348:946–50.
6. Bewley S, Cockburn J. Responding to fear of childbirth. Lancet 2002;359:2128–9.
7. Saisto T, Salmela-Aro K, Nurmi J-E, Kononen T, Halmesmaki E. A randomized controlled trial of intervention in fear of childbirth. Obstet Gynecol 2001;98:820–6.
8. Morrison J, MacKenzie IZ. Cesarean section on demand. Semin Perinatol 2003;27:20–33.
9. Chervenak FA, McCullough LB. An ethically justified algorithm for offering, recommending, and performing cesarean delivery and its application in managed care practice. Obstet Gynecol 1996;87:302–5.

Patient Testing

In the practice of medicine, clinical evaluation is enhanced by a broad range of tests. Recommendations to patients about testing should be based on current medical knowledge, a concern for the patient's best interests, and mutual consultation. Patient testing embodies many scientific and human ideals. From an ethical perspective, the most important principles involve a trusting patient–physician relationship, a focus on the benefits the patient may derive from testing, and an appreciation that patients make choices about their medical care.

Rapid technological development and the need to consider legal and sociocultural factors as well as medical knowledge have increased the complexity of the decision-making process. The physician often is in the position of ordering tests—human immunodeficiency virus (HIV) or genetic markers, for example—that may, unlike a urinalysis or a hemogram, have a profound nonmedical effect on the patient, her partner, her family, and society in general. This new level of complexity requires the specification of both medical and ethical guidelines for decisions about patient testing. This chapter provides ethical guidance for decisions about ordering tests, counseling patients, and reporting results.

Ordering Tests

- *The physician and the patient have a shared responsibility.* The quality of medical care improves when there is clear communication and mutual understanding between physician and patient. It is the responsibility of the obstetrician–gynecologist to communicate effectively and to develop skills that promote a patient–physician relationship characterized by trust and honesty. Similarly, it is the responsibility of the patient to provide accurate information about her lifestyle, health habits, sexu-

al practices, and religious and cultural beliefs when these factors may affect medical judgment. In decisions about testing, physicians should be guided by scientific knowledge. Care must be taken to avoid subjective assumptions based on bias that could affect the appropriateness of testing.

- *Testing should be performed primarily for the benefit of the patient.* Testing at the request of third parties—partners, health care providers, members of the patient's extended family, employers, or health insurers—is justifiable only when the patient or her valid proxy understands the potential risks and benefits and gives consent. Examples of this type of testing include genetic tests to assist family members with reproductive decisions and HIV tests to fulfill conditions for the purchase of life insurance.

- *The decision to offer or to withhold a test should not be made solely on the basis of a physician's assumptions about the patient's expected response to test results.* Prejudgments about a patient's wishes regarding fetal abnormalities, for example, should not preclude her being offered prenatal testing. The patient should join with the physician in deciding the amount of diagnostic information that is appropriate for making intelligent choices about preventive care and treatment options. The physician is not, however, ethically obligated to perform every test a patient requests.

- *The patient must be informed prospectively about policies regarding use of information and legal requirements.* The patient must be told what will be communicated, to whom, and the potential implications of reporting the information. If, for example, a patient is aware that a specific hospital has a policy of posting HIV test results in the medical record and access to the results may be available, she may choose instead to use an anonymous testing procedure available through

Previously published as Committee Opinion 159, October 1995

another laboratory. In some situations, reporting of results is mandated by law. Physicians should be familiar with the laws regarding mandatory testing and reporting requirements in their own jurisdictions.

- *The physician and patient should discuss concerns about cost containment and reimbursement.* The mutual goal of physician and patient should be to avoid both undertesting and overtesting. Contemporary focus on the economics of health care has created worries for both physician and patient about access to care, limitations to testing, appropriateness of utilization, and the impact of financial constraints on quality of care. Open communication about cost concerns is the best way to alleviate suspicion and to promote trust.

Pretest and Posttest Counseling

- *Testing that may have multiple medical or psychosocial consequences requires specific counseling.* The extent of counseling beneficial to each patient will vary depending on the individual and on the implications inherent in the potential test results. With simple tests like urinalysis, it is sufficient to provide information about the nature and purpose of the test and how the results will guide management. Tests that may have multiple medical or psychosocial ramifications require comprehensive explanation of the process, the goals, and the implications. Counseling can be appropriate for genetic testing and maternal toxicology assays, for example, because of the potential for psychologic, social, and economic impact. Testing for HIV or genetic testing may limit future insurance coverage. A positive toxicology screen could result in the removal of children from the household.
- *Both pretest and posttest counseling facilitate women's access to appropriate health care.* Pretest counseling includes both medical considerations and issues such as the availability of emotional support while waiting for test results. Posttest counseling offers an opportunity to provide access to resource networks and community-based services.
- *Referral may be needed for comprehensive counseling.* If time constraints or lack of technical expertise make it difficult to offer comprehensive counseling in a particular practice, appropriate options include either 1) referral to a specialized center for both counseling and testing, or 2) refer-

ral for counseling only, with return to the original physician for testing and medical follow-up.

Confidentiality and the Reporting of Test Results

- *Information ordinarily may not be revealed without the patient's express consent.* Physicians have an obligation to be familiar with federal privacy protection legislation (Health Insurance Portability and Accountability Act [HIPAA]). Guidance is provided here for the ethical duty to maintain confidentiality. Maintaining confidentiality is intrinsic to respect for patient autonomy and permits the free exchange of information that is relevant to medical decision making. Situations may arise, however, in which a physician has competing obligations: protecting the patient's confidentiality or disclosing test results to prevent harm to a third party. In these situations, every avenue of communication should first be explored in discussions with the patient about rights and responsibilities. Consultation with an institutional ethics committee or a medical ethics specialist may be helpful in weighing benefits and harms of disclosure. Legal advice may be prudent.
- *A violation of confidentiality may be ethically justified as a last resort.* A violation of confidentiality may be justifiable only when legally required or when all of the following conditions have been met: 1) there is a high probability of harm to a third party, 2) the potential harm is a serious one, 3) the information communicated can be used to prevent harm, and 4) greater good will result from breaking confidentiality than from maintaining it.

Conclusion

In addition to establishing a diagnosis, testing provides opportunities to educate, inform, and advise. The ethical principles of respect for autonomy (patient choice) and beneficence (concern for the patient's best interests) should guide the testing, counseling, and reporting process. Clear and ample communication fosters trust, facilitates access to services, and improves the quality of medical care.

Suggested Reading

American College of Medical Genetics, American College of Obstetricians and Gynecologists. Preconception and prenatal carrier screening for cystic fibrosis: clinical and laboratory guidelines. Washington, DC: ACOG; 2001.

American College of Obstetricians and Gynecologists. HIPAA privacy manual. 2nd ed. Washington, DC: ACOG; 2003.

Davis DS. Genetic dilemmas: reproductive technology, parental choices, and children's futures. New York (NY): Routledge; 2000.

McGowan R. Beyond the disorder: one parent's reflection on genetic counselling. J Med Ethics 1999;25:195–9.

Nelson RM, Botkin JR, Kodish ED, Levetown M, Truman JT, Wilfond BS, et al. Ethical issues with genetic testing in pediatrics. Pediatrics 2001;107:1451–5.

Secretary's Advisory Committee on Genetic Testing. Enhancing the oversight of genetic tests: recommendations of the SACGT. Bethesda (MD): SACGT; 2000. Available at http://www4.od.nih.gov/oba/sacgt/reports/oversight-report.pdf. Retrieved July 18, 2003.

Human Immunodeficiency Virus

As of 1999, nearly 120,000 American women had been reported as having acquired immunodeficiency syndrome (AIDS), approximately 16.5% of affected adult Americans (1). In addition, more than 33,000 American women have been reported as being infected with the human immunodeficiency virus (HIV) in the 34 areas that report HIV infection, representing approximately 17% of Americans whose infection has been reported (1). Women represent the subgroup with the fastest rate of increase in HIV infections. Most of these women are not aware of their positive serostatus (2). Diagnosis of HIV in women usually is made during prenatal antibody screening or in conjunction with screening for sexually transmitted diseases (STDs). Because most of the women newly identified as HIV positive during pregnancy are not aware that they have been exposed to HIV infection and do not consider themselves to be at risk, universal testing is preferable to targeted, risk-based testing (3). This lack of awareness of risk, accompanied by generally low levels of accurate information about HIV, has led some to question the need for pretest counseling in hopes of reducing the barriers to universal testing. The tension between competing goals for HIV testing—to test broadly to treat women and protect fetuses and to offer thorough counseling to protect maternal autonomy and a woman's right to participate in decision making—has sparked considerable debate.

Because HIV infection is detected through prenatal and STD screening, it is likely that an obstetrician–gynecologist will provide care for an infected woman. This chapter provides guidance to obstetrician–gynecologists regarding ethical issues associated with HIV pretest counseling and consent and disclosure of positive test results. It also outlines re-

Previously published as Committee Opinion 255, April 2001; content revised January 2004

sponsibilities related to providing patient care to infected women, access of affected couples to assisted reproductive technology (ART), and the responsibilities of the HIV-infected health care professional.

Human Immunodeficiency Virus Antibody Counseling and Testing

Prenatal Counseling and Testing

The major ethical principles that must be considered when formulating policies for prenatal HIV antibody counseling and testing include maternal autonomy, confidentiality, justice, protection of vulnerable individuals, and beneficence to both the pregnant woman and her fetus. Three major prenatal HIV counseling and testing strategies have been endorsed by different public health and public policy officials, all with a goal of universal testing: 1) voluntary testing with counseling regarding risks and benefits (with or without signed consent); 2) testing with patient notification and right of refusal; and 3) mandatory testing with no right of refusal.

Voluntary Testing with Counseling. Voluntary testing with counseling is the strategy most consistent with respect for patient autonomy for both pregnant and nonpregnant women. Under this option, physicians should be prepared to provide both pretest and posttest counseling. Some physicians may perform such counseling themselves, whereas others may prefer to refer the patient for counseling and testing. In addition to medical information, such counseling should include information regarding potential uses of test information and legal requirements pertaining to the release of information. Patients should be told what information will be communicated and to whom and the possible implications of reporting the information. Having these facts will aid patients in making the decision whether to undergo antibody testing.

Testing with Patient Notification and Right of Refusal. The second strategy, HIV testing with patient notification and right of refusal, was recommended by the Institute of Medicine to address clinicians' concerns that pretest counseling and informed consent mandates for routine voluntary testing in pregnancy were too time consuming and, thus, reduced the likelihood of testing being offered (4). Recent evidence suggests that this strategy may be acceptable to as many as 70% of pregnant women (5). The testing with notification strategy removes the requirement for pretest counseling and informed consent except in those states where these provisions are required by law. Under the notification strategy, physicians must inform all patients that routine prenatal blood work will include HIV antibody testing and inform them of their right to refuse this test. The goal of this strategy is to make HIV antibody testing less cumbersome and more likely to be performed by incorporating it into the routine battery of prenatal tests. If testing barriers are reduced, more doctors may offer testing, which may lead to the identification and treatment of more infected women and their fetuses. This testing strategy aims to balance competing ethical considerations. On the one hand, personal freedom (maternal autonomy) is diminished, and there are social risks to HIV-positive women from disclosure of HIV status. On the other hand, medical and social benefits to both the woman and her fetus and a reduced burden to society may result from treatment-associated reduction of perinatal HIV infection (maternal and fetal beneficence). Although some welcome the Institute of Medicine-sponsored policy for testing with notification for pregnant women for the potential benefits it confers, others have raised concerns about: 1) the inequality inherent in having one standard for nonpregnant women and a separate, less autonomous standard for pregnant women; 2) the potential for testing with notification to degenerate into notification after testing in today's busy, pressured practice environment; and 3) the lack of evidence that dispensing with pretest counseling and informed consent actually will increase the number of tests performed.

Testing with patient notification is an ethically acceptable prenatal testing strategy provided that the patient is given the option to refuse testing. If this testing strategy is elected, a clinician must notify the patient that HIV testing is routinely performed as a part of the antenatal testing protocol and inform her

that she has the right to refuse the test. Refusal of testing should not have an adverse effect on the care the patient receives or lead to denial of care. This guarantee of a right to test refusal ensures that maternal autonomy is not completely abridged in the quest to achieve a difficult-to-reach public health goal (ie, the elimination of perinatal transmission of HIV infection).

The American College of Obstetricians and Gynecologists has taken the position of qualified support for this strategy, with the important addition that Fellows be encouraged to include counseling as a routine part of care, but not as a prerequisite for, or barrier to, prenatal HIV testing (6). Similarly, the American Medical Association has recommended that universal HIV testing of all pregnant women, with patient notification of the right of refusal, should be a routine component of prenatal care and adds that basic counseling on HIV prevention and treatment also should be provided to the patient, consistent with the principles of informed consent (7). Accordingly, physicians should be prepared to provide both pretest and posttest counseling.

Mandatory Testing Without Right of Refusal. The third option, mandatory testing with no right of refusal, only can be achieved by law. Mandatory prenatal testing strategies are problematic because they abridge maternal autonomy. In addition, the public health objective of this strategy, universal testing, has been accomplished in certain populations by other ethically sound testing strategies (8). The rationale for mandatory testing is that it would be a more efficient way of achieving universal testing. Advocates support this strategy based on the greatest good for the greatest number, a belief that the potential benefit to the pregnant woman and the fetus overrides maternal burden, and a desire to reduce economic costs to society by preventing infection of the fetus. Supporters of mandatory testing believe that these benefits justify abridging maternal autonomy. Mandatory prenatal HIV testing is difficult to define and to defend ethically and has few precedents in modern medicine. Advocates of testing without notification cite the reduction of congenital syphilis as an example of the effectiveness of mandatory prenatal testing. This analogy is inappropriate, however, because syphilis is treated by a short course of antibiotics, and treatment of HIV infection is far more complex and problematic. There is no scientific evidence, as yet, that either testing with notification or mandatory testing without right of refusal will increase the number of HIV tests performed.

Human immunodeficiency virus testing is not without risk for a pregnant woman. If the test result is positive, she faces the possibility of being ostracized by her family, friends, and community. In addition, there is potential for job discrimination, loss of health insurance, and loss of housing. If a woman decides to accept treatment, complex drug treatment regimens and their side effects constitute a significant burden (9). Mandatory testing may compromise the ability to form an effective physician–patient relationship at the very time when this relationship is critical to the success of treatment. Although it is treatment, not testing, that confers the benefit to the woman, to the fetus, and to society, mandatory treatment for HIV has been rejected by ethicists and clinicians alike. Accordingly, mandatory prenatal HIV testing should be rejected for the same reasons. Ultimately, it is a short-sighted and limited strategy.

Counseling and Testing of Nonpregnant Women

Nonpregnancy-related HIV counseling and testing occurs most commonly in conjunction with screening for STDs in both inpatient and outpatient settings. Women should be informed that they are being screened for HIV infection, and they should be informed of the local policies regarding use and distribution of the test information. Full informed consent should precede testing in these settings, and the ramifications of a positive test result should be discussed fully before antibody testing is performed. All women should be afforded the option of refusing testing. Refusal of testing should not have an adverse effect on the care the patient receives or lead to denial of care. Women who receive positive test results should receive posttest counseling, including options for therapy and follow-up. Women who receive negative test results but have lifestyle factors that place them at high risk for contracting infection should be offered risk reduction counseling.

Human Immunodeficiency Virus Reporting and Partner Notification

The clinician providing care for an HIV-infected woman has important responsibilities concerning disclosure of the patient's serostatus. Clinicians providing health care should be aware of and respect legal requirements regarding confidentiality and disclosure of HIV-related clinical information. A breach of confidentiality may be required by mandatory reporting requirements.

Situations may arise in which clinicians have competing obligations: protecting the patient's confidentiality and disclosing test results to prevent substantial harm to a third party. In these situations, the clinician should first educate the patient about her rights and responsibilities and encourage her to inform any third parties involved. Consultation with an institutional ethics committee, a medical ethics specialist, or an attorney may be helpful in deciding whether or not to disclose her HIV status. Confidentiality should not be breached solely because of perceived risk to health care workers. Health care workers should rely on strict observance of standard precautions to minimize risk. The patient's HIV serostatus, however, should be transmitted to other health care professionals to ensure optimal medical management.

A breach of confidentiality may be ethically justified for purposes of partner notification when 1) there is a high probability of harm to the partner, 2) the potential harm is a serious one, 3) the information communicated can be used to prevent harm, and 4) greater good will result from breaking confidentiality rather than maintaining it. When a breach of confidence is contemplated, however, practitioners should weigh the potential harm to the patient and to society at large. Negative consequences of breaking confidentiality may include:

- Personal risks to the individual whose confidence is breached, such as serious implications for the patient's relationship with family and friends, the threat of discrimination in employment and housing, domestic violence, and the impact on family members

- Loss of patient trust, which may reduce the physician's ability to communicate effectively and provide services

- A ripple effect among cohorts of women that may deter other women at risk from accepting testing and have a serious negative impact on the educational efforts that lie at the heart of attempts to reduce the spread of disease

If, on balance, a breach of confidence is deemed necessary, practitioners should consider whether the goal of maintaining patient privacy would be better served by personal communication with the individual placed at risk by the patient's seropositivity or by notification of local public health authorities. In some areas, anonymous notification of sexual contacts is possible through local or state departments of health.

Because individuals are living longer as a direct result of therapeutic advances with HIV and data on AIDS no longer offer a complete picture of the epidemic or its impact on the health care system, the Centers for Disease Control and Prevention has endorsed name-based reporting of HIV infection, generating intense debate among public health officials. Proponents of name-based reporting cite the benefits of accurately tracking the epidemic to plan for current and future HIV-related health care expenditures and facilitating voluntary partner notification. Opponents fear that name-based reporting will discourage patients from undergoing HIV antibody testing. Both supporters and opponents of name-based reporting agree that safeguards must be in place to protect patient confidentiality. Participating in name-based reporting to public health authorities is ethically acceptable provided that confidentiality is protected.

Health Care Professionals' Obligation To Provide Care

It is unethical for an obstetrician–gynecologist to refuse to accept a patient or to continue care for a patient solely because she is or is thought to be seropositive for HIV. Refusing to provide care to HIV-infected women for fear of contracting HIV infection or simply as a practice preference is unreasonable, unscientific, and unethical.

Epidemiologic studies have shown that the risk of HIV transmission from patient to health care professional is exceedingly low and is related to needle stick or intraoperative injury or to potentially infectious fluid that comes in contact with a mucous membrane (10). Most contacts between health care professionals and HIV-infected women occur, however, during routine obstetric and gynecologic care. Health care practitioners should observe standard precautions with all patients to minimize skin, mucous membrane, and percutaneous exposure to blood and body fluids to protect against a variety of pathogens, including HIV.

There are physicians who require HIV testing as a precondition for providing prenatal care or performing a surgical procedure. There are other physicians who may require a blood sample that can be tested for HIV in the event that they may be inadvertently exposed to the patient's blood or body fluid in the course of providing care. Although consent usually is forthcoming, some women refuse HIV testing as a precondition of receiving care. In the event of patient refusal to be tested, the clinician should treat the patient as though she is HIV positive. A physician may have the legal right to transfer care to another qualified physician based on such refusal. However, such a transfer would be ethically debatable. It clearly would be unethical if it reflects an unwillingness to care for an HIV-infected patient or may have an adverse effect on the care the patient may receive.

Not only do health care professionals who fail to provide care to HIV-infected women because of personal practice preferences violate professional ethical standards, they also place an undue burden on their professional colleagues who are willing to provide health care to these women. Finally, the public has invested both personally and economically in the education of health care professionals (11) and appropriately expects that health care practitioners will not discriminate based on diagnosis, provided that the patient's care falls within their scope of practice. Physicians should demonstrate integrity, compassion, honesty, and empathy. Failure to provide care to a woman solely because she is infected with HIV violates these fundamental characteristics. As with any other patient, it is acceptable, however, to refer HIV-infected women for care that the physician is not competent to provide, for patient convenience, or for financial reasons.

Assisted Reproductive Technology

There is an emerging consensus that ART should be offered to some couples in which one or both partners are infected with HIV, and it has been widely stated that now there is an ethical obligation to provide ART to such couples, consistent with respect for both autonomy and beneficence (12, 13). Those who support providing these services to this population cite 3 major reasons. First, therapeutic improvements in the management of HIV infection have enhanced both quality and length of life for HIV-positive individuals. Second, advances in prenatal therapy have substantially reduced the risk of mother-to-infant HIV transmission. Third, current ART methods will reduce transmission of HIV from an infected partner to an uninfected partner.

Those who oppose offering these technologies to HIV-infected couples cite 2 major objections: 1) uncertain long-term parental prognosis and 2) the continuing risk of maternal-to-fetal HIV transmission. The ethical underpinning of this opposition is that it is not felt to be in the best interest of the child to be born to a parent who may not be available for continuing childrearing. In addition, the risk of maternal-to-child transmission places the child at risk of acquiring a highly debilitating illness.

Requests for ART by HIV-infected couples probably will increase. The pool of infected individuals with stable illness and with or without infertility is growing. These individuals are becoming aware of the low risk of maternal-to-infant HIV transmission with appropriate treatment and may want to attempt pregnancy. Moreover, when a couple in which one partner is HIV positive elects to conceive a child through ART rather than unprotected sexual intercourse, it may in fact reduce the transmission of HIV between partners.

Assisted reproductive technology should not be denied to HIV-infected couples solely on the basis of their positive serostatus. Offering this technology to infected individuals is consistent with balancing respect for autonomy with fetal beneficence. Also, there is precedent for offering ART to individuals with other chronic and potentially lethal diseases. This field is an emerging one and is changing rapidly. Patients should be cared for by practitioners who have current knowledge and expertise in this field.

Health Care Practitioners Infected With Human Immunodeficiency Virus

In making decisions about patient care, health care practitioners who are infected with HIV should adhere to the fundamental professional obligation to avoid harm to patients. Physicians who have reason to believe that they have been at significant risk of being infected should be tested voluntarily for HIV for the protection of their patients. The physician as a patient is entitled to the same rights to privacy and confidentiality as any other patient.

Although the risk of clinician-to-patient transmission is extremely low, all infected physicians must make a decision as to which procedures they can continue to perform safely. This decision primarily will depend on the particular surgical technique involved and also on the physician's level of expertise and medical condition, including mental status. The clinician's decision should be made in consultation with a personal physician and may possibly involve such other responsible individuals as the chief of the department, the hospital's director of infectious diseases, the chief of the medical staff, or a specialized advisory panel. If physicians avoid procedures that place patients at risk of harm, they

have no obligation to inform the patient of their positive HIV serostatus.

Physicians who are infected with HIV should follow standard precautions, including the appropriate use of hand-washing, protective barriers, and care in the use and disposal of needles and other sharp instruments. They also should comply with current guidelines for disinfection and sterilization of reusable devices used in invasive procedures.

References

1. Perinatally aquired AIDS, 1985–1998, United States. Centers for Disease Control and Prevention. HIV AIDS Surveill Rep 1999;11(2):1–44.
2. Gwinn M, Wortley PM. Epidemiology of HIV infection in women and newborns. Clin Obstet Gynecol 1996;39: 292–304.
3. Donegan SP, Steger KA, Recla L, Hoff RS, Werner BG, Rice PA, et al. Seroprevalence of human immunodeficiency virus in parturients at Boston City Hospital: implications for public health and obstetric practice. Am J Obstet Gynecol 1992;167:622–9.
4. Institute of Medicine. Reducing the odds: preventing perinatal transmission of HIV in the United States. Washington, DC: National Academy Press; 1999.
5. Carusi D, Learman LA, Posner SF. Human immunodeficiency virus test refusal in pregnancy: a challenge to voluntary testing. Obstet Gynecol 1998;91:540–5.
6. American Academy of Pediatrics, American College of Obstetricians and Gynecologists. Joint statement on human immunodeficiency virus screening. ACOG Statement of Policy 75. Elk Grove Village, (IL): AAP; Washington, DC: ACOG; 1999.
7. American Medical Association, Council on Scientific Affairs. Universal, routine screening of pregnant women for HIV infection. CSA report 1 (I-01). Chicago (IL): AMA, 2002. Available at http://www.ama-assn.org/ama/pub/article/2036-6983.html. Retrieved July 28, 2003.
8. Prenatal discussion of HIV testing and maternal HIV testing—14 states, 1996–1997. MMWR Morb Mortal Wkly Rep 1999;48:401–4.
9. Strathdee SA, Palepu A, Cornelisse PG, Yip B, O'Shaughnessy MV, Montaner JS, et al. Barriers to use of free antiretroviral therapy in injection drug users. JAMA 1998;280:547–9.
10. Public Health Service guidelines for the management of health-care worker exposures to HIV and recommendations for postexposure prophylaxis. Centers for Disease Control and Prevention. MMWR Recomm Rep 1998; 47(RR-7):1–33.
11. Beauchamp TL, Childress JF. Principles of biomedical ethics. 5th ed. New York (NY): Oxford University Press; 2001.
12. Anderson DJ. Assisted reproduction for couples infected with the human immunodeficiency virus type 1 [editorial]. Fertil Steril 1999;72:592–4.
13. Minkoff H, Santoro N. Ethical considerations in the treatment of infertility in women with human immunodeficiency virus infection. N Engl J Med 2000;342:1748–50.

Patient Choice in the Maternal–Fetal Relationship

The maternal–fetal relationship is unique in medicine because of the complete physiologic dependence of the fetus on the pregnant woman and because both the fetus and the woman are regarded as patients of the obstetrician. Moreover, therapeutic access to the fetus occurs through the body and person of the pregnant woman, who may experience negative effects from interventions designed to benefit the fetus. The welfare of the fetus is of the utmost importance to almost all pregnant women. However, there are 2 areas in which maternal and fetal interest can be apparently divergent: 1) the pregnant woman may refuse a diagnostic procedure, medical therapy, or a surgical procedure intended to enhance or preserve fetal well-being; and 2) the pregnant woman's behavior may be deleterious to the fetus.

Medicine aims to foster the greatest benefit with the least risk. Risks and benefits, however, may be valued differently by the pregnant woman and the obstetrician, creating the potential for disagreement. When the fetus may be in danger, the woman often is asked to consent to diagnostic procedures or therapy for the sole or primary benefit of the fetus. Examples of this are a cesarean delivery for fetal indications, intrauterine fetal transfusion for isoimmunization, or zidovudine to prevent the perinatal transmission of human immunodeficiency virus (HIV) infection. Also, a pregnant woman may be entreated to modify her behavior in the interest of fetal well-being and almost always in her own interest as well. For example, the obstetrician may suggest a smoking cessation program or modifications of diet for diabetes or phenylketonuria. The obstetrician's response to a patient's unwillingness to cooperate with medical advice in these situations should be to convey clearly the reasons for the recommen-

Previously published as Committee Opinion 214, April 1999; content revised January 2004

dations to the pregnant woman, examine the barriers to change along with her, and encourage the development of health-promoting behavior. The obstetrician should be aware of state and local laws and regulations that may require reporting certain maternal behaviors to designated authorities.

In interactions with a woman who appears to resist following medical advice that might improve her health or that of her fetus, the obstetrician must keep in mind that medical knowledge has limitations and medical judgment is fallible. Existing methods for detection of nonreassuring fetal status are not always reliable indicators of poor outcome, and there often is insufficient evidence for risk determination or risk–benefit evaluation for the fetus. In addition, expected benefits for the fetus cannot always be achieved. Similarly, in situations, such as cesarean delivery, in which there is statistically a low degree of maternal risk, occasional serious maternal complications may occur. Because of the inability to determine with certainty when a situation is harmful to the fetus and to guarantee that the pregnant woman will not be harmed by the medical intervention, great care should be exercised to present a balanced evaluation of expected outcomes for both parties. The obstetrician's recommendations must be made in clear, understandable terms, taking into consideration the patient's age, educational level, cultural background, and language ability. Family members, friends of the patient, social workers, religious counselors, interpreters, and other caregivers may help the patient clarify her position if she chooses to confide in them. Consultation with an institutional ethics committee or other institutional resource may provide a useful forum for discussion and potential resolution of the problem.

The pregnant woman may decide that the risk of a recommended treatment is greater than she wishes to accept, or she may doubt the benefit of the treatment for either herself or the fetus. When a competent patient chooses not to comply with the recommended treatment after all reasonable attempts to explain and persuade have been exhausted, the obstetrician has 3 choices. One choice is to respect the patient's autonomy and not proceed with the recommended intervention regardless of the consequences. A second choice is to offer the patient the option of obtaining medical care from another individual before an emergency situation arises that might put the pregnant woman and the caregiver in unresolvable conflict. A caregiver would exercise this alternative if unwilling to comply with a patient's expressed decision about medical intervention or nonintervention, because of the caregiver's opinion that such actions might adversely affect the fetus. Patients should be encouraged to discuss fully their concerns and choices early in the course of prenatal care so that appropriate action may be taken before a crisis occurs. A third option, exercised on rare occasions, is to request involvement of the court. The choice among these unpleasant options will depend on the urgency of the clinical circumstances, the potential consequences for both the pregnant woman and the fetus, and the reliability of predictions of such consequences.

Three ethical principles may be helpful in choosing among these options: 1) respect for autonomy—the obligation of the physician to respect the right of the pregnant woman to choose or refuse recommended treatment; 2) beneficence—the obligation of the physician to promote the pregnant woman's well-being as well as that of the fetus and the obligation of the pregnant woman to promote the well-being of her fetus; and 3) justice—the obligation to treat similar people similarly. Abiding by the patient's autonomous decision will provide the best care for the pregnant woman and the fetus in most circumstances. Occasionally, a woman's autonomous decision will seem not to promote beneficence-based obligations (of the woman or the physician) to the fetus. In this situation, when there is insufficient time to obtain transfer of care, the obstetrician must respect the patient's autonomy, continue to care for the pregnant woman, and not intervene against the patient's wishes, regardless of the consequences. Such action may subordinate the caregiver's personal ethic to his or her professional obligation to respect the patient's autonomy.

Another important principle that should be considered is the principle of justice, which requires that individuals (in this case, both pregnant and nonpregnant patients) be treated fairly. Those who argue against court-ordered intervention invoke the principle of justice, arguing that generally, one individual cannot be compelled to undergo medical treatment, particularly surgery, to benefit another. For example, an individual cannot be compelled to donate an organ or bone marrow to save the life of another, even if the potential recipient is the individual's child. It follows, then, that a woman's right to refuse invasive medical treatment that would benefit another should not be diminished because she is pregnant. Justice requires that pregnant and nonpregnant individuals should be afforded similar rights.

Nonetheless, the application of principle-based ethics to issues in perinatology has been criticized for its tendency to emphasize the divergent rather than the shared interests of the pregnant woman and fetus, ignore women's forms of moral reasoning, and at times reinforce social and racial inequality. Given that most court-ordered interventions (seemingly justified by the principle of beneficence) have been sought against poor women of color, some have suggested that principle-based ethics fails to account for the ways that socioeconomic factors affect maternal–fetal decision making. An alternative model proposes that moral obligations be considered with regard to the woman and fetus not as separate or separable entities, but as a maternal–fetal unit situated in a particular social, political, and cultural context. Thus, clinicians faced with ethical dilemmas in perinatology should attempt to understand pregnant women's decisions within their broad social networks and communities, examine how clinicians' own standpoints influence their ethical decision making, and determine whether clinicians' conclusions reinforce existing gender, class, or racial inequality.

In the past 2 decades, health care providers have infrequently resorted to court-ordered authorization of intervention that is against a pregnant patient's wishes. These decisions have been challenged from both a legal and ethical perspective. In a landmark case, *In re AC*, the DC Court of Appeals overturned a previous court-ordered authorization of cesarean delivery, saying that if a competent pregnant woman makes an informed decision, "her wishes will control in virtually all cases." Furthermore, the court stated that "we do not quite foreclose the possibility that a conflicting state interest may be so compelling that the patients's wishes must yield, but we anticipate that such cases will be extremely rare and truly exceptional."

The Committee on Ethics agrees that court-ordered intervention against the wishes of a pregnant woman is rarely if ever acceptable. If health care providers contemplate going to court for authorization of interventions that are against pregnant patients' wishes, the legal and ethical precedents outlined here should be considered and the following criteria should be met: 1) there is high probability of serious harm to the fetus in respecting the patient's decision; 2) there is high probability that the recommended treatment will prevent or substantially reduce harm to the fetus; 3) there are no comparably effective, less-intrusive options to prevent harm to the fetus; and 4) there is high probability that the recommended treatment also benefits the pregnant woman or that the risks to the pregnant woman are relatively small. These criteria must be weighed against the following 3 factors: 1) a woman is wronged and may be harmed, whether physically, psychologically, or spiritually, when her autonomy is violated; 2) the patient's subsequent loss of trust in the health care system may reduce the health care provider's ability to help her and may deter others from seeking care; and 3) there may be other social costs associated with this violation of individual liberty (see also "End-of-Life Decision Making" in Part II).

Even in the presence of a court order authorizing intervention, the use of physical force against a resistant, competent woman is not justified. The use of force will substantially increase the risk to the woman, thereby diminishing the ethical justification of such therapy.

Conclusions

1. The maternal–fetal relationship is unique because it involves the obligation of the physician to respect the autonomy of the pregnant woman, in the context of the obstetrician's beneficence-based obligations to the pregnant woman and her fetus, the pregnant woman's beneficence-based obligations to her fetus, and considerations of justice regarding the treatment of pregnant women. Every reasonable effort should be made to protect the fetus, but the pregnant woman's autonomy should be respected.
2. The vast majority of pregnant women are willing to assume significant risk for the welfare of their fetuses. Problems arise when potentially benefi-

cial advice is rejected. The role of the obstetrician should be one of an informed educator and counselor, weighing the risks and benefits to both patients as well as realizing that tests, judgments, and decisions are fallible. Obstetricians should consider the social and cultural context in which these decisions are made and question whether their ethical judgments reinforce gender, class, or racial inequality. Consultation with others, including an institutional ethics committee, should be sought when appropriate to aid the pregnant woman and obstetrician in resolving the conflict. The use of the courts to resolve these conflicts is warranted only in extraordinary circumstances.

3. Obstetricians should refrain from performing procedures that are unwanted by a pregnant woman. The use of judicial authority to implement treatment regimens to protect the fetus violates the pregnant woman's autonomy and should be avoided. In addition to wronging the pregnant woman, appeal to judicial authority may lead to undesirable societal consequences, such as the criminalization of noncompliance with medical recommendations.

Bibliography

Adams SF, Mahowald MB, Gallagher J. Refusal of treatment during pregnancy. Clin Perinatol 2003;30:127–40, vii–viii.

Draper H. Women, forced caesareans and antenatal responsibilities. J Med Ethics 1996;22:327–33.

Harris LH. Rethinking maternal–fetal conflict: gender and equality in perinatal ethics. Obstet Gynecol 2000;96:786–91.

In re A.C., 573 A.2d 1235 (D.C. App. 1990)

Johnsen D. A new threat to pregnant women's autonomy. Hastings Cent Rep 1987;17(4):33–40.

Kolder VE, Gallagher J, Parsons MT. Court-ordered obstetrical interventions. N Engl J Med 1987;316:1192–6.

Murray TH. Moral obligations to the not-yet-born child. In: The worth of a child. Berkeley (CA): The University of California Press; 1996. p. 96–114.

Robertson JA. Legal issues in fetal therapy. Semin Perinatol 1985;9:136–42.

Robertson JA, Schulman JD. Pregnancy and prenatal harm to offspring: the case of mothers with PKU. Hastings Cen Rep 1987;17(4):23–33.

Tauer CA. Lives at stake: how to respond to a woman's refusal of cesarean surgery when she risks losing her child or her life. Health Prog 1992;73:18, 20–7.

Sex Selection

Sex selection is the practice of using medical techniques to choose the sex of offspring. Patients may request sex selection for different reasons. Medical indications include the prevention of sex-linked genetic disorders. In addition, there are a variety of social, economic, cultural, and personal reasons for selecting the sex of children. In cultures in which males are more highly valued than females, sex selection has been practiced to ensure that offspring will be male.

Currently, reliable techniques for selecting sex are limited to postfertilization methods. Postfertilization methods include techniques used during pregnancy as well as techniques used in assisted reproduction before the transfer of embryos fertilized in vitro (see "Preembryo Research" in Part III). Recent attention, however, has focused on preconception techniques, particularly flow cytometry separation of X-bearing and Y-bearing spermatozoa before intrauterine insemination or in vitro fertilization (IVF).

This chapter discusses various ethical considerations and arguments relevant to both prefertilization and postfertilization techniques for sex selection. It also provides recommendations for health care professionals who may be asked to participate in sex selection.

Indications

The principal medical indication for sex selection is known or suspected risk of sex-linked genetic disorders. For example, 50% of males born to women who carry the gene for hemophilia will have this condition. By identifying the sex of the preimplantation embryo or fetus, a woman can learn whether or

Previously published as Committee Opinion 177, November 1996; content revised January 2004

not the 50% risk of hemophilia applies, and she can receive appropriate prenatal counseling. To ensure that surviving offspring will not have this condition, some women at risk for transmitting hemophilia choose to abort male fetuses or choose not to transfer male embryos. Where the marker or gene for a sex-linked genetic disorder is known, selection on the basis of direct identification of affected embryos or fetuses, rather than on the basis of sex, is possible. Direct identification has the advantage of avoiding the possibility of aborting an unaffected fetus or deciding not to transfer unaffected embryos. Despite the increased ability to identify genes and markers, in certain situations, sex determination is the only current method of identifying embryos or fetuses potentially affected with sex-linked disorders [1].

Inevitably, identification of sex occurs whenever karyotyping is performed. When medical indications for genetic karyotyping do not require information about sex chromosomes, the prospective parent(s) may elect not to be told the sex of the fetus.

Other reasons sex selection is requested are personal, social, or cultural in nature. For example, the prospective parent(s) may prefer that an only or first-born child be of a certain sex or may desire a balance of sexes in the completed family [2].

Methods

There are a variety of techniques for sex identification and selection. These include techniques used before fertilization, after fertilization but before embryo transfer, and, most frequently, after implantation.

Prefertilization

Techniques for sex selection before fertilization include timing sexual intercourse and using various methods for separating X-bearing and Y-bearing

sperm (3–10). No current techniques for prefertilization sex selection have been shown to be reliable.
Recent attention, however, has focused on flow
cytometry separation of X-bearing and Y-bearing
spermatozoa as a method of enriching sperm populations for insemination. This technique allows
heavier X-bearing sperm to be separated, and therefore selection of females alone may be achieved with
increased probability (11). More research is needed
to determine whether any of these techniques can be
endorsed in terms of reliability or safety.

Postfertilization and Pretransfer

Assisted reproductive technologies, such as IVF,
make possible biopsy of one or more cells from a
developing embryo at the cleavage or blastocyst
stage (12). Sex selection is therefore possible in conjunction with these reproductive technologies.

Postimplantation

After implantation of a fertilized egg, karyotyping of
fetal cells will provide information about fetal sex.
This presents patients with the option of terminating
pregnancies for the purpose of sex selection.

Ethical Positions of Other Organizations

Many organizations have issued statements concerning the ethics of provider participation in sex selection. The ethics committee of the American Society
for Reproductive Medicine (formerly, the American
Fertility Society) maintains that the use of preconception sex selection by preimplantation genetic
diagnosis for nonmedical reasons is ethically problematic and "should be discouraged" (13). However,
it issued a statement in 2001 that if prefertilization techniques, particularly flow cytometry for
sperm sorting, were demonstrated to be safe and
efficacious, these techniques would be ethically
permissible for family balancing (14). Because
preimplantation genetic diagnosis is physically more
burdensome and necessarily involves the destruction
and discarding of embryos, it was not considered
similarly permissible for family balancing (15).

Both the President's Commission for the Study
of Ethical Problems in Medicine and Biomedical
and Behavioral Research and the Programme of
Action adopted by the United Nations International
Conference on Population and Development opposed
the use of sex selection techniques for any nonmedical reason (16, 17). The latter group urges govern-
ments of all nations "to take necessary measures to
prevent...prenatal sex selection."

The International Federation of Gynecology and
Obstetrics rejects sex selection when it is used as a
tool for sex discrimination. It supports preconceptional sex selection when it is used to avoid sex-
linked genetic disorders (18).

The United Kingdom's Human Fertilisation and
Embryology Authority released new guidance on
preimplantation genetic diagnosis in 2003 (19). The
guidance, which replaces interim guidance issued in
1999, states that "centres may not use any information derived from tests on an embryo, or any material removed from it or from the gametes that produced it, to select embryos of a particular sex for
non-medical reasons."

Discussion

Medical Testing Not Expressly for the Purpose of Sex Selection

Providers may participate unknowingly in sex selection when information about the sex of a fetus
results from a medical procedure performed for
some other purpose. For example, when a procedure
is done to rule out medical disorders in the fetus,
the sex of a fetus may become known and may
be used for sex selection without the provider's
knowledge.

The Committee on Ethics maintains that when a
medical procedure is done for a purpose other than
obtaining information about the sex of a fetus but
will reveal the fetus's sex, this information should
not be withheld from the pregnant woman who
requests it. This is because this information legally
and ethically belongs to the patient (20–22). As a
consequence, it might be difficult for providers to
avoid the possibility of unwittingly participating in
sex selection. To minimize the possibility that they
will unknowingly participate in sex selection, physicians should foster open communication with
patients aimed at clarifying patients' goals. Although
providers may not ethically withhold medical information from patients who request it, they are not
obligated to perform an abortion, or other medical
procedure, to select fetal sex. Physicians should
explicitly inform patients, in advance when possible,
if they are unwilling to perform specific medical
procedures that patients might request.

Medical Testing Expressly for the Purpose of Sex Selection

With regard to medical procedures performed for the
express purpose of selecting the sex of a fetus, the

following 3 potential ethical positions are outlined to facilitate discussion:

Position 1: Never participate in sex selection. Providers may never ethically perform medical procedures with the intended purpose of sex selection.

Position 2: Participate in sex selection when medically indicated. Providers may ethically perform medical procedures with the intended purpose of preventing sex-linked genetic disorders.

Position 3: Participate in sex selection whenever requested. Providers may ethically perform medical procedures for the purpose of sex selection whenever the patient requests such procedures.

The committee rejects, as too restrictive, the position that sex selection techniques are always unethical (position 1). The committee supports, as ethically permissible, the practice of offering patients procedures for the purpose of preventing serious sex-linked genetic diseases (position 2). For example, it supports offering patients using assisted reproductive techniques the option of preimplantation genetic diagnosis for identification of male sex chromosomes if patients are at risk for transmitting Duchenne's muscular dystrophy. This position is consistent with the stance of equality between the sexes because it does not imply that the sex of a child itself makes that child more or less valuable.

The committee rejects the position that sex selection should be performed on demand (position 3), because this position may reflect and encourage sex discrimination. In most societies where sex selection is widely practiced, families prefer male offspring. Although this preference sometimes has an economic rationale, such as the financial support or physical labor male offspring traditionally provide or the financial liability associated with female offspring, it also reflects the belief that males are inherently more valuable than females. There exists a relationship between women's social, legal, and economic status and the tendency of women and men to prefer sons: generally, son-preference increases as women's social status decreases (23). Where systematic preferences for a particular sex dominate, this suggests the need to address underlying inequalities between the sexes.

The committee shares the concern expressed by the President's Commission for the Study of Ethical Problems in Medicine and Biomedical and Behavioral Research, the United Nations, and the International Federation of Gynecology and Obstetrics that sex selection can be motivated by and reinforce the devaluation of women. The committee supports the ethical principle of equality between the sexes.

Some argue that sex selection techniques are ethically justified when used for reasons other than disease prevention. For example, sex selection may be requested to achieve a "balance" in a family in which all current children are the same sex and a child of the opposite sex is desired (13). To achieve this goal, couples may request 1) sperm sorting by flow cytometry to enhance the probability of achieving a pregnancy of a particular sex, although these techniques are considered experimental; 2) transferring only embryos of one sex in assisted reproduction; 3) reducing, based on sex, the number of fetuses in a multifetal pregnancy; or 4) aborting fetuses that are not of the desired sex. In these situations, individual parents may consistently judge sex selection to be an important personal or family goal and, at the same time, reject the idea that children of one sex are inherently more valuable than children of another sex.

Although this stance is, in principle, consistent with the principle of equality between the sexes, it nonetheless raises ethical concerns. First, it often is impossible to ascertain patients' true motives for requesting sex selection procedures. For example, patients who want to abort female fetuses because they value male offspring more than female offspring, or because they want their first-born children to be male, would be unlikely to espouse such beliefs openly if they thought this would lead physicians to deny their requests. Second, even when sex selection is requested for nonsexist reasons, the very idea of preferring a child of a particular sex may be interpreted as condoning sexist values and, hence, create a climate in which sex discrimination can more easily flourish. Even preconceptional techniques of sex selection may encourage such a climate. The use of flow cytometry is experimental, and preliminary reports indicate that achievement of a female fetus is not guaranteed. Misconception about the accuracy of this evolving technology coupled with a strong preference for a child of a particular sex may lead couples to terminate a pregnancy of the "undesired" sex. The committee concludes that nonmedical uses of sex selection techniques have the potential to undermine equality between the sexes; moreover, this ethical objection arises irrespective of the timing of selection (ie, preconception or postconception) or the stage of development of the embryo or fetus.

Conclusion

The committee accepts, as ethically permissible, the practice of sex selection to prevent sex-linked genetic disorders. The committee opposes meeting requests for sex selection that are based on the belief that offspring of a certain sex are inherently more valuable. The committee opposes meeting requests for sex selection for personal and family reasons, such as family balancing, because of the concern that such requests may ultimately support sexist practices.

Medical techniques intended for other purposes have the potential of being used by patients for sex selection without the provider's knowledge or consent. Because patients are entitled to obtain personal medical information, including information about the sex of their fetus, it will sometimes be impossible for health professionals to avoid unwitting participation in sex selection.

In this chapter, the committee has sought to assist physicians and other health care providers facing requests from patients for sex selection by calling attention to relevant ethical considerations, affirming the value of equality between the sexes, and emphasizing that individual providers are never ethically required to participate in sex selection.

References

1. Winston RM, Handyside AH. New challenges in human in vitro fertilization. Science 1993;260:932–6.
2. Young R. The ethics of selecting for fetal sex. Ballieres Clin Obstet Gynaecol 1991;5:575–90.
3. Gray RH. Natural family planning and sex selection: fact or fiction? Am J Obstet Gynecol 1991;165:1982–4.
4. Shushan A, Schenker JG. Prenatal sex determination and selection. Hum Reprod 1993;8:1545–9.
5. Pyrzak R. Separation of X- and Y-bearing human spermatozoa using albumin gradients. Hum Reprod 1994;9:1788–90.
6. Check JH, Zavos PM, Katsoff D, Kiefer D. Effects of Percoll discontinuous density gradients vs SpermPrep II vs Sephadex G-50 gel infiltration on semen parameters. Arch Androl 1993;31:69–73.
7. Martin RH. Human sex pre-selection by sperm manipulation. Hum Reprod 1994;9:1790–1.
8. Check JH, Kastoff D. A prospective study to evaluate the efficacy of modified swim-up preparation for male sex selection. Hum Reprod 1993;8:211–4.
9. Check JH, Katsoff D, Kozak J, Lurie D. Effect of swim-up, Percoll, and Sephadex sperm separation methods on the hypo-osmotic swelling test. Hum Reprod 1992;7:109–11.
10. Wang HX, Flaherty SP, Swann NJ, Matthews CD. Discontinuous Percoll gradients enrich X-bearing human spermatozoa: a study using double-label fluorescence in-situ hybridization. Hum Reprod 1994;9:1265–70.
11. Fugger EF, Black SH, Keyvanfar K, Schulman JD. Births of normal daughters after MicroSort sperm separation and intrauterine insemination, in-vitro fertilization, or intracytoplasmic sperm injection. Hum Reprod 1998;13:2367–70.
12. Hardy K, Martin KL, Leese HJ, Winston RM, Handyside AH. Human preimplantation development in vitro is not adversely affected by biopsy at the 8-cell stage. Hum Reprod 1990;5:708–14.
13. Sex selection and preimplantation genetic diagnosis. The Ethics Committee of the American Society for Reproductive Medicine. Fertil Steril 1999;72:595–8.
14. Ethics Committee of the American Society for Reproductive Medicine. Preconception gender selection for nonmedical reasons. Fertil Steril 2001;75(5):861–4.
15. Robertson J. Sex selection: final word from the ASRM Ethics Committee on the use of PGD. Hastings Cent Rep 2002;32(2):6.
16. President's Commission for the Study of Ethical Problems in Medicine and Biomedical and Behavioral Research. Screening and counseling for genetic conditions: a report on the ethical, social, and legal implications of genetic screening, counseling, and education programs. Washington, DC: Government Printing Office; 1983.
17. United Nations. Gender equality, equity and empowerment of women. In: Population and development: programme of action adopted at the International Conference on Population and Development; 1994 Sept 5–13; Cairo. New York (NY): UN; 1995. p. 17–21.
18. International Federation of Gynecology and Obstetrics (FIGO). Sex selection. In: Recommendations on ethical issues in obstetrics and gynecology by the FIGO Committee for the Ethical Aspects of Human Reproduction and Women's Health. London: FIGO; 2000. p. 8–9.
19. Human Fertilisation and Embryology Authority. HFEA guidance on preimplantation genetic testing. London: HFEA; 2003. Available at: http://www.hfea.gov.uk/forClinics/archived/chair_letters/03032003/CH0304AnnexA.pdf. Retrieved July 30, 2003.
20. Jonsen AR, Siegler M, Winslade WJ. Clinical ethics: a practical approach to ethical decisions in clinical medicine. 5th ed. New York (NY): McGraw-Hill; 2002.
21. American Hospital Association. A patient's bill of rights. Chicago (IL): AHA; 1992. Available at: www.hospitalconnect.com/aha/about/pbillofrights.html. Retrieved July 30, 2003.
22. American Medical Association. Patient information. In: Code of medical ethics: current opinions with annotations. Chicago (IL); 2002. p. 217–9.
23. Warren MA. The prospect of sex selection. In: Gendercide: the implications of sex selection. Totowa (NJ): Rowman and Allanheld; 1985. p. 6–31.

Multifetal Pregnancy Reduction

The ethical issues surrounding the use and consequences of reproductive technologies are highly complex, and no one position reflects the variety of opinions within the membership of the American College of Obstetricians and Gynecologists. The purpose of this chapter is to review the ethical issues involved in multifetal pregnancy reduction. For the purposes of this document, multifetal pregnancy reduction is defined as a first-trimester or early second-trimester procedure for termination of 1 or more fetuses in a multifetal pregnancy, to increase the chances of survival of the remaining fetuses and decrease long-term morbidity for the delivered infants (1).

To many, the ethical issues involved in multifetal pregnancy reduction are somewhat different from the issues involved in abortion, as discussed in the "Analysis" section later in this chapter. Although no physicians need participate in any activities that they find morally unacceptable, all physicians should be aware of the medical and ethical issues in these complex situations and be prepared to respond in a professional, ethical manner to patient requests for information and procedures.

Background

Spontaneous occurrences of multifetal pregnancies always have been a medical problem. More recently, increased use of potent ovulation-induction drugs and assisted reproductive technology (ART), such as in vitro fertilization (IVF), have been effective in the treatment of infertility but subsequently also have increased the risk of multifetal pregnancy (2). Thousands of patients previously unable to have children have been assisted to achieve conception. In a small

Previously published as Committee Opinion 215, April 1999; content revised January 2004

percentage of these patients, the resultant pregnancy has involved more than 2 fetuses, thereby creating potentially serious problems (2–7). There is widespread agreement that the risks of perinatal morbidity and mortality and maternal morbidity increase with the number of fetuses. Recent reports have shown improving outcomes with multifetal pregnancies, but the risks are still significant (7).

Prevention

The first approach to this problem is or should be prevention. It might be argued that the problem is best remedied by discontinuing technologic assistance to reproduction. On the one hand, this approach discounts the major benefits that ART offers to patients and suggests an unwarranted coercive restriction on parental choice and autonomy. On the other hand, the association of an increased rate of multifetal pregnancies with infertility treatment deserves serious attention. Some multifetal pregnancies will inevitably occur despite the best of intentions, knowledge, skill, and equipment, but it is essential that those providing infertility treatment exercise a high degree of diligence to minimize the problem.

Both ovulation induction alone and IVF contribute to high-order multiple births (more than 2). In 1977, 43.3% of all births of triplets or greater were the result of ART (ie, IVF) and 38.2% were the result of the use of ovulation drugs (6). In 1996, the order was reversed; 40.4% of births of triplets or greater were the result of ovulation drugs, whereas 38.7% were the result of ART (6). According to the Centers for Disease Control and Prevention, 3,117 infants were born in triplet or higher-order deliveries after ART treatment in 2000. Similar data are not available for ovulation induction cycles (8).

Ovulation induction with gonadotropin cycles in which ultrasound imaging demonstrates the presence of many mature follicles, each capable of releasing an ovum, presents a difficult decision on whether to give human chorionic gonadotropin (hCG) to induce ovulation. If an hCG injection is withheld, the patient will have spent considerable time and emotional and financial resources for a nonovulatory cycle. Yet, if hCG is given to trigger ovulation, a high-order multifetal pregnancy may result. Attempts have been made to develop criteria for withholding hCG (eg, more than 6 large follicles or estradiol levels >1,500 pg/mL). However, a large study showed that the occurrence of high-order multifetal pregnancies after gonadotropin therapy increases with higher estradiol levels but cannot be reliably predicted by the number of mature follicles on ultrasound (9). The authors concluded that adherence to criteria for withholding hCG will not prevent high-order multiple births and that better criteria cannot easily be established. They suggest that the use of treatment protocols with less-intensive stimulation of the ovaries may reduce the incidence of high-order multifetal pregnancies, but only to a limited extent and at the expense of pregnancy rates. Alternative approaches when many follicles are present would be conversion of the gonadotropin cycle to an IVF cycle or selective aspiration of the supernumerary follicles (10).

In ART, there may be pressures to be successful because of both prospective parents' and programs' interests. Direct costs for IVF cycles are many times higher than those for ovulation induction alone with gonadotropins. Because ovulation induction with gonadotropins may be more likely to be covered by insurance, patients who choose to undergo IVF may be paying for treatment out of pocket and this may add pressure to achieve pregnancy on the first attempt. In addition, IVF programs face public scrutiny not faced by programs that offer only ovulation induction. Although success rates for individual IVF programs are public information, published by the Centers for Disease Control and Prevention, similar reporting is not done for ovulation induction alone (2). As the number of embryos transferred increases, program success rates may increase, but so does the risk of a multifetal pregnancy (11, 12).

The physician who makes decisions about the circumstances for triggering ovulation or guidelines for embryo transfer must, as in any medical situation, place the best interests of the patient and the future child or children at the center of the risk–benefit equation. In some countries, such as England, where ART is centrally regulated, limitations are placed on the number of embryos that can be transferred and subsequently fewer multifetal pregnancies result.

In the United States, the decision is left to individual physicians and programs. In almost all cases, it is preferable to terminate a gonadotropin cycle used for ovulation induction alone or limit the number of embryos to be transferred in IVF to prevent a situation in which patients and physicians will have to consider fetal reduction. The Practice Committee of the American Society for Reproductive Medicine has issued a report suggesting prognosis-dependent guidelines for limiting the number of embryos to be transferred. These guidelines limit risk while allowing individualization of patient care for optimal results (13). Multifetal pregnancy reduction should be viewed as a response to a consequence of ovulation induction that cannot always be avoided; it should not be a routinely accepted treatment for an iatrogenic problem.

The ultimate goal in prevention is to significantly reduce the likelihood that any multifetal pregnancy will occur, including twins. This will require patients, physicians, and payors to support a culture in which IVF may replace gonadotropin-only therapy in treatment algorithms. When IVF is performed, the eventual goal in the future may be to transfer only the embryo with the greatest chance for growth and implantation.

Counseling

As with all medical care, counseling for treatment of infertility should incorporate discussions of risks, benefits, and treatment alternatives, including the option for no treatment. Counseling should be considered an ongoing process, beginning before treatment decisions are made and continuing throughout the patient's care. The risks of certain treatments of infertility include, but are not limited to, the occurrence of multifetal pregnancy, with its associated risks of spontaneous abortion, preterm labor and delivery, and neonatal morbidity and mortality. The informed consent process must include information about the potential for multifetal pregnancy and associated maternal risks, such as prolonged hospitalization, antepartum bleeding, postpartum hemorrhage, hypertensive diseases of pregnancy, and an increased rate of cesarean delivery.

It also is the responsibility of the physician to inform the patient that fetal reduction as a response to multifetal pregnancy has inherent medical risks to the remaining fetuses, such as a reported pregnancy loss of 4.5–7.6% for triplet-to-twin reduction in large multicenter samples (14, 15). Reports of lower birth weights for twins reduced from triplets also are of concern (16–18), although other reports have suggested that reduction from triplets or quadruplets to twins is associated with an outcome as good as with an unreduced twin gestation (15, 19–22). Nonetheless, patients should not be given the impression that multifetal pregnancies are without problems because fetal reduction is available.

Patients struggle with the ethical and emotional issues of fetal reduction. In 2 postdelivery informational surveys of couples who had undergone multifetal pregnancy reduction (23, 24), more than one half of the small samples of respondents reported that they did not understand the procedure or its consequences fully at the time of fetal reduction (25). A significant proportion reported still feeling guilt (24, 25), even though they believed that the procedure was necessary. Many infertility patients have unrealistic ideas about the outcomes for high-order multifetal pregnancies (25–27) that leave them unprepared for feelings of loss and grief at the time of a reduction procedure. However, in studies that used standard psychologic tests to assess the emotional state of patients after multifetal pregnancy reduction, serious long-term psychologic sequelae were not identified; depression scores for women who did not carry to term after reduction were similar to scores for a control group of women who experienced a spontaneous abortion but no fetal reduction (28, 29).

The report that 93% of patients who decided to proceed with fetal reduction would make that decision again despite their experience of stress and sadness is somewhat reassuring, but the number of patients studied, either by self-report survey or by standard psychologic measures, was quite small (n=91) (29). The ethical issues that this option involves should be discussed with patients before the initiation of any treatment that could increase the risk of multifetal pregnancy. Although patients should be encouraged to examine their feelings about these risks and options at the onset, the counseling process should encourage them to continue this assessment at appropriate points in the treatment process (30).

Options

In the presence of an already established multifetal pregnancy, the options are inevitably difficult. No choice is without potential consequences, and the potential benefits must be carefully weighed against the potential harms. There are 3 options in multifetal pregnancies:

1. Abort the entire pregnancy (all the fetuses).
2. Continue the pregnancy (all the fetuses).
3. Perform multifetal pregnancy reduction on 1 or more of the fetuses.

The first option involves aborting the entire multifetal pregnancy. However, for some patients, aborting the pregnancy is not an acceptable option. For other patients who may have achieved pregnancy after infertility treatment, this option may be considered the least desirable.

The second option is attempting to carry the multifetal pregnancy to term. However, the risks of perinatal and maternal morbidity and mortality increase directly with the number of fetuses (9). These risks include losing all the fetuses or having some survive with permanent impairment as a consequence of extreme preterm birth. The assessment of what constitutes "significant risk" varies among patients and physicians and is therefore not amenable to uniform definition. Physicians should respect their patients' conclusions about which risks are acceptable and which are too high.

The third option in multifetal pregnancies is multifetal pregnancy reduction. The technique brings about the demise of 1 or more fetuses with the intent to allow continuation of the pregnancy, resulting in the delivery of fewer infants with lower risks of preterm birth, morbidity, and mortality. Although this procedure is successful in most cases, it may raise some unsettling ethical concerns. There is a complex interrelationship between the intention to reduce the morbidity of a smaller number of surviving fetuses and the intentional sacrifice of others that demands an ethical as well as medical assessment of the relative benefits and risks of multifetal pregnancy reduction. What follows is an attempt to outline such an assessment, with the understanding that each case ultimately must be examined on its own merits.

Analysis

Many would argue that there are differences between the ethical analyses involved in multifetal pregnancy reduction and elective abortion because the intent is different. A woman has an elective abortion because, for many complex and varied reasons, she does not wish or feels unable to have a child. In contrast, an infertility patient who has a multifetal pregnancy undergoes fetal reduction precisely because she does wish to bear a child. The patient and her physician may conclude that fetal reduction is the preferred way to continue her pregnancy. For some individuals, the primary intention justifying fetal reduction may be the life and well-being of the fetuses that do survive and continue to develop. For others, it is unethical to terminate an apparently healthy fetus, even for the sake of the survival or well-being of other fetuses in the pregnancy.

Some individuals who believe that abortion is generally unacceptable find multifetal pregnancy reduction to be justified ethically when the risks of carrying the pregnancy are considerable and could be reduced if the number of fetuses were fewer. Individual patients will evaluate varying degrees of risk differently. As advances in maternal–fetal and neonatal medicine continue, the risk of extreme preterm birth is expected to decrease. The issues of patient choice and physician participation and consultation need to be analyzed on a case-by-case basis.

Summary

Although physicians may choose not to participate in multifetal pregnancy reduction, they should be knowledgeable about this procedure and be prepared to react in a professional and ethical manner to patient requests for information or services or both. The first approach to the problem of multifetal pregnancies should be prevention. Although fetal reduction will be ethically acceptable to many as a response to an unforeseen and unavoidable contingency, in almost all cases, it is preferable to terminate a gonadotropin cycle or limit the number of embryos to be transferred to prevent a situation in which the patient and physician need to consider fetal reduction. Counseling for treatment of infertility should include the risks of multifetal pregnancy, and the ethical issues surrounding fetal reduction should be discussed with patients before the initiation of any treatment that could increase the risk of multifetal pregnancy.

References

1. Berkowitz RL, Lynch L. Selective reduction: an unfortunate misnomer. Obstet Gynecol 1990;75:873–4.
2. Centers for Disease Control and Prevention. 2000 Assisted reproductive technology success rates: national summary and fertility clinic reports. Atlanta (GA): CDC; 2002.
3. Evans MI, Fletcher JC, Zador IE, Newton BW, Quigg MH, Struyk CD. Selective first-trimester termination in octuplet and quadruplet pregnancies: clinical and ethical issues. Obstet Gynecol 1988;71:289–96.
4. Berkowitz RL, Lynch L, Chitkara U, Wilkins IA, Mehalek KE, Alvarez E. Selective reduction of multifetal pregnancies in the first trimester. N Engl J Med 1988;318:1043–7.
5. Wapner RJ, Davis GH, Johnson A, Weinblatt VJ, Fischer RL, Jackson LG, et al. Selective reduction of multifetal pregnancies. Lancet 1990;335:90–3.
6. Contribution of assisted reproduction technology and ovulation-inducing drugs to triplet and higher-order multiple births—United States, 1980–1997. MMWR Morb Mortal Wkly Rep 2000;49:535–8.
7. Jones HW, Schnorr JA. Multiple pregnancies: a call for action [editorial]. Fertil Steril 2001;75:11–3.
8. Wright VC, Schieve LA, Reynolds MA, Jeng G. Assisted reproductive technology surveillance—United States, 2000. MMWR Surveill Summ 2003;52:1–16.
9. Gleicher N, Oleske DM, Tur-Kaspa I, Vidali A, Karande V. Reducing the risk of high-order multiple pregnancy after ovarian stimulation with gonadotropins. N Engl J Med 2000;343:2–7.
10. ESHRE Task Force on Ethics and Law. 6. Ethical issues related to multiple pregnancies in medically assisted procreation. Hum Reprod 2003;18:1976–9.
11. Martin PM, Welch HG. Probabilities for singleton and multiple pregnancies after in vitro fertilization. Fertil Steril 1998;70:478–81.
12. Templeton A, Morris JK. Reducing the risk of multiple births by transfer of two embryos after in vitro fertilization. N Engl J Med 1998;339:573–7.
13. American Society for Reproductive Medicine. Guidelines on number of embryos transferred. ASRM Practice Committee Report. Birmingham (AL): ASRM; 1999.
14. Evans MI, Dommergues M, Wapner RJ, Goldberg JD, Lynch L, Zador IE, et al. International, collaborative experience of 1789 patients having multifetal pregnancy reduction: a plateauing of risks and outcomes. J Soc Gynecol Investig 1996;3:23–6.
15. Evans MI, Berkowitz RL, Wapner RJ, Carpenter RJ, Goldberg JD, Ayoub MA, et al. Improvement in outcomes of multifetal pregnancy reduction with increased experience. Am J Obstet Gynecol 2001;184:97–103.
16. Silver RK, Helfland BT, Russell TL, Ragin A, Sholl JS, MacGregor SN. Multifetal reduction increases the risk of preterm delivery and fetal growth restriction in twins: a case-control study. Fertil Steril 1997;67:30–3.
17. Groutz A, Yovel I, Amit A, Yaron Y, Azem F, Lessing JB. Pregnancy outcome after multifetal pregnancy reduction to twins compared with spontaneously conceived twins. Hum Reprod 1996;11:1334–6.
18. Depp R, Macones GA, Rosenn MF, Turzo E, Wapner RJ, Weinblatt VJ. Multifetal pregnancy reduction: evaluation of fetal growth in the remaining twins. Am J Obstet Gynecol 1996;174:1233–8; discussion 1238–40.
19. Papageorghiou AT, Liao AW, Skentou C, Sebire NJ, Nicolaides KH. Trichorionic triplet pregnancies at 10–14 weeks: outcome after embryo reduction compared to expectant management. J Matern Fetal Neonatal Med 2002;11:307–12.

20. Miller VL, Ransom SB, Shalhoub A, Sokol RJ, Evans MI. Multifetal pregnancy reduction: perinatal and fiscal outcomes. Am J Obstet Gynecol 2000;182:1575–80.

21. Yaron Y, Bryant-Greenwood PK, Dave N, Moldenhauer JS, Kramer RL, Johnson MP, et al. Multifetal pregnancy reductions of triplets to twins: comparison with nonreduced triplets and twins. Am J Obstet Gynecol 1999; 180:1268–71.

22. Torok O, Lapinski R, Salafia CM, Bernasko J, Berkowitz RL. Multifetal pregnancy reduction is not associated with an increased risk of intrauterine growth restriction, except for very-high-order multiples. Am J Obstet Gynecol 1998; 179:221–5.

23. Kanhai HH, de Haan M, van Zanten LA, Geerinck-Vercammen C, van der Ploeg HM, Gravenhorst JB. Follow-up of pregnancies, infants and families after multifetal pregnancy reduction. Fertil Steril 1994;62:955–9.

24. Vauthier-Brouzes D, Lefebvre G. Selective reduction in multifetal pregnancies: technical and psychological aspects. Fertil Steril 1992;57:1012–6.

25. Garel M, Starck C, Blondel B, Lefebvre G, Vauthier-Brouzes D, Zorn JR. Psychological effects of embryonal reduction. From the decision making to 4 months after delivery [French]. J Gynecol Obstet Biol Reprod (Paris) 1995;24:119–26.

26. Gleicher N, Campbell DP, Chan CL, Karande V, Rao R, Balin M, et al. The desire for multiple births in couples with infertility problems contradicts present practice patterns. Hum Reprod 1995;10:1079–84.

27. Goldfarb J, Kinzer DJ, Boyle M, Kurit D. Attitudes of in vitro fertilization and intrauterine insemination couples toward multiple gestation pregnancy and multifetal pregnancy reduction. Fertil Steril 1996;65:815–20.

28. McKinney M, Downey J, Timor-Tritsch I. The psychological effects of multifetal pregnancy reduction. Fertil Steril 1995;64:51–61.

29. Schreiner-Engel P, Walther VN, Mindes J, Lynch L, Berkowitz RL. First-trimester multifetal pregnancy reduction: acute and persistent psychologic reactions. Am J Obstet Gynecol 1995;172:541–7.

30. Zaner RM, Boehm FH, Hill GA. Selective termination in multiple pregnancies: ethical considerations. Fertil Steril 1990;54:203–5.

Adoption

Adoption is a commonly used alternative strategy for family building. Although adoption is not a medical event per se, obstetrician–gynecologists may find themselves at the center of adoption issues because of their expertise in the assessment and management of infertility, pregnancy, and childbirth. There are several specific roles that the obstetrician–gynecologist may be asked to assume regarding adoption. Physicians commonly provide information, advice, and counsel, and they refer birth parents and prospective adoptive parents to adoption agencies. They also may be asked to link or match pregnant women with families desiring adoption. Frequently, they are asked to provide information about prospective parents to adoption agencies. In each of these roles, it is important that obstetrician–gynecologists consider the rights, responsibilities, and safety of all concerned parties: the child, the birth parents, the prospective adoptive parents, and themselves.

Six principles have historically guided adoption practices (1):

1. Consent of the birth mother was a necessary precondition for adoption, whereas presumed waiver of consent by absent birth fathers has been routine.

2. The purpose of adoption was to serve the child's best interests by placement with suitable adoptive parents.

3. Adoption practices were based on the principle of gratuitous transfer, and financial transactions suggestive of purchase of a child were prohibited.

4. Relationships with adoptive parents were expected to substitute entirely for relationships with biologic parents.

5. Relinquishing birth mothers and adopting parents were assured that their confidentiality and anonymity would be protected.

6. Adoptive relationships were presumed to be permanent once they were finalized in court.

These principles currently are undergoing redefinition and reconsideration. Physicians should be aware of the following new trends in adoption practices:

1. There is increased emphasis on the rights of biologic fathers and reluctance to use a waiver process to release a child for adoption when the biologic father cannot be located.

2. Concepts of suitability of adoptive parents and the best interests of the child are undergoing reconsideration.

3. The present environment of competition for adoptive infants may lead to inducements in the form of subsidies for medical care and other support, making the gratuitous nature of adoption less clear and free of financial conflict.

4. Proponents of openness in adoption argue that adoption should include complementary relationships with birth parents. Even in a closed adoption, the adopted child and adoptive parents need to have access to relevant genetic and medical information about the biologic parents.

5. It is no longer possible to guarantee absolute confidentiality to either birth or adoptive parents. Most states have laws that give adopted individuals access to their birth records.

6. Adoption can no longer be considered to be permanent in every case, because situations have arisen in which adoptive relationships were terminated by adoptive parents, biologic parents, or adopted children after a final adoption decree had been granted.

Previously published as Committee Opinion 194, November 2001; content revised January 2004

The resulting lack of clarity about both ethical issues and legal consequences may create a potentially hazardous situation for physicians. In the following sections, the different roles that the obstetrician–gynecologist may be asked to play in adoption are described. Ethical concerns are discussed, and safeguards are proposed.

Education

The physician's role in education is to ensure that adoption is introduced into the description of alternatives for women with unwanted pregnancies and for potential adoptive parents. Physicians have a responsibility to provide information about adoption to all patients with unwanted pregnancies and to all patients with infertility concerns (2). Fact sheets distributed by the American College of Obstetricians and Gynecologists (3) and the American Society for Reproductive Medicine (4) support this educational role. Physicians have an obligation to present alternatives fairly, regardless of personal values and beliefs. They should not advocate for or against relinquishment or adoption. Nor should they avoid discussing these issues when they are appropriate to the patient's situation. This position is consistent with the right of adults to the information required to make fully informed decisions. It also is consistent with the ethical obligation to promote what is good for the patient. These obligations can be met, for some patients, by placing literature about adoption in the reception area, thereby validating adoption as a legitimate, respected choice. A lengthy counseling session, in which the risks and benefits of adoption are weighed against other alternatives, may be indicated for other patients.

Physicians may have both positive and negative personal biases about adoption for various reasons. For example, physicians who have chosen the adoption alternative as their own method of family building may present this option either positively or negatively, depending on their individual experiences. Physicians would do well to disclose their potential sources of bias, and take special care to uphold the principle of respect for patient autonomy.

Physicians also should ensure that financial incentives do not bias the presentation of information about adoption. For example, physicians must be especially careful to offer information about adoption to patients with established infertility because money accrues to a gynecologist from the treatment of infertile patients, and these fees may cease with a decision to adopt rather than pursue further treatment.

Advice and Counseling

The physician's role in advising and counseling patients is to assist those for whom adoption may be appropriate in making a decision that is right for them. Patients often turn to their physicians and say, "Doctor, what do you think I should do?" Women experiencing unwanted pregnancy or infertility are vulnerable, facing confusing and painful situations. The physician is a caregiver, trained to solve problems and help patients feel better. The temptation to advocate for a specific position can be great. It may seem to the physician that the obvious solution for a young woman who is unemployed is to relinquish her child or for an infertile couple who are reasonable candidates for in vitro fertilization to pursue that option before considering adoption.

It is appropriate for physicians to give advice on medical matters. This is an essential part of the physician–patient relationship and an expert role for which physicians are trained. Patients count on the guidance of physicians for medical decisions. Adoption, however, is only tangentially a medical matter, and few physicians are expert in this field. Furthermore, for the physician, the particular encounter with an individual patient or couple, no matter how compelling, occurs only during a finite point in time. The patients will be living with the lifelong consequences of these decisions. Therefore, physicians who provide advice and counsel, unless they are truly expert in the field of adoption, should guard against advocating for a particular action. The best counsel will permit the involved parties to explore their options fully and make a decision that arises out of their own beliefs, values, needs, and circumstances.

Referrals

The physician's role in referrals is to identify appropriate resources. Physicians often may best fulfill their obligations to patients through referral to other professionals who have the appropriate skills and expertise to address the difficult issues raised by adoption. For example, referral to a mental health professional for short-term counseling provides an opportunity for both birth and prospective adoptive parents to explore their emotional reactions and the ways that different alternatives may affect their lives. Some patients may feel more comfortable having a discussion of this type with someone who is not involved with their ongoing medical care.

When an obstetrician–gynecologist makes a medical referral, there is an ethical obligation to investigate the skills and credentials of the consultant. The same responsibility for protecting the patient's best interests pertains to psychologic and social referral resources. As a starting point, there are many sources of information available to assist physicians in developing their own lists of referral alternatives (see "Resources" at the end of this chapter). In addition, local hospitals maintain referral rosters.

Screening

When authorized by patients, the physicians' role in screening is to provide appropriate information to screening agencies regarding patients' qualifications as prospective parents for an adoptive child. Physicians often are asked by patients to fill out forms requesting information about their mental, psychologic, and medical suitability as prospective adoptive parents. Physicians are bound by ethical precepts to be truthful, to act in their patients' best interests, and to protect their patients' confidentiality. Adoption agencies, however, give precedence to the needs and interests of adoptive children.

Difficult situations may arise. A patient may request, for example, that a physician not reveal to the agency the extent of her chronic illness and its potential effect on her life expectancy. Although a physician may wish to advocate for a patient, there is an obligation to be truthful and to let patients know what can and cannot be said.

Many agency forms request the treating physician to certify that the individual or couple is fit to parent. If the physician of record believes that he or she does not have enough information to make a judgment, the agency may count that as evidence against the couple. The physician must be honest and speak accurately to the information that is available. The best approach is for the physician to disclose to the patient what will be written in the report, followed by frank discussion with the patient of the potential impact of the report.

Limits to the Physician's Role

If asked to serve as a broker in an independent adoption, the physician's role is to refer the patient to an appropriate agency or adoption resource. Among all the roles that physicians play in adoption, that of a broker is perhaps the most hazardous because of ethical issues related to undue influence, competing obligations, and lack of expertise.

Although both birth parents and prospective adoptive parents generally view the adoption agreement as a binding promise, patients may find themselves unable or unwilling to fulfill that promise after delivery of the child. The pregnant woman who agreed to relinquish her child may have done so in good faith with the best knowledge available to her at that time. She may not know what that promise really means or if she can really do what she agreed to until she has given birth to this child, held it, and experienced the extent of loss. The couple who agreed to accept a child may regret that decision and feel unable to keep their part of the agreement if, for example, the child is born with serious medical problems. For these and similar reasons, no adoption agreement is legally binding before the birth of the child.

If a physician has acted as a broker and the adoption agreement falls through, he or she will be aware of the loss experienced by the other party, may feel responsible, and may be tempted to use the power of the patient–physician relationship to influence the patient to fulfill the original promise. The physician's ability to provide current or future medical care for this patient may be compromised by these events.

Brokering adoptions is properly the role of an independent authority or agency, which is in a position to protect the interests of all involved parties—the child, the birth parents, and the adoptive parents. For these reasons, many hospitals have bylaws prohibiting staff physicians from direct involvement as adoption brokers. Physicians should avoid matching prospective adoptive parents with women who have unwanted pregnancies and should instead refer patients to agencies or other adoption resources, when available. Physicians should receive only the usual compensation for medical and counseling services. Referral fees and other arrangements for financial gain beyond usual fees for clinical services are inappropriate.

When physicians also are prospective adoptive parents, there may be a temptation to adopt an infant from one of their own patients. This arrangement is unethical. It contravenes principles of fairness to other potential parents and takes advantage of patients' highly vulnerable situations.

Summary

The adoption field is evolving, and the issues are complex. Obstetrician–gynecologists can play helpful and effective roles in adoption as educators and advisers. Adoption should be presented fairly, along with other options, to all those who might benefit. Physicians can be excellent sources of information, can assist in weighing risks and benefits, and can provide emotional support. When authorized by patients to fill out forms for adoption agencies, physicians should do so truthfully, with full disclosure to patients of what they intend to say.

Physicians should involve themselves in counseling and screening roles with great care because potential exists for unintended misuse of the physician–patient relationship. Patient confidentiality, patient autonomy, and the principle of the patient's best interest may be compromised by subtle or blatant conflicts of interest. Physicians are advised to delegate to an independent authority all responsibility for matching pregnant women with prospective adoptive parents.

References

1. Hollinger JH. Adoption law. Future Child 1993;3:43–61.
2. Kaunitz AM, Grimes DA, Kaunitz KK. A physician's guide to adoption. JAMA 1987;258:3537–41.
3. American College of Obstetricians and Gynecologists. Pregnancy choices: raising the baby, adoption, and abortion. ACOG Patient Education Pamphlet AP102. Washington, DC: ACOG; 2002.
4. American Society for Reproductive Medicine. Patient's fact sheet: adoption. Birmingham (AL): ASRM; 2003.

Resources

Arcus D. Adoption. In: The Gale encyclopedia of psychology, 2nd ed. Detroit (MI): Gale Group; 2001. p. 15–9.

National Adoption Information Clearinghouse (330 C St, SW, Washington, DC 20447; telephone: (703) 352-3488 or 888-251-0075; http://www.calib.com/naic/), a comprehensive resource on all aspects of adoption, is a service of the U.S. Department of Health and Human Services.

Perspectives Press (PO Box 90318, Indianapolis, IN 46290-0318; telephone: (317) 872-3055; www.perspectivespress.com) concentrates on issues related to adoption.

Resolve (1310 Broadway, Somerville, MA 02144; telephone: 888-623-0744; www.resolve.org), the organization for infertile couples, maintains a directory of nationally and locally recognized and accredited organizations and individuals who provide adoption support.

Surrogate Motherhood

Although the practice of surrogate motherhood has become more common since the American College of Obstetricians and Gynecologists (ACOG) issued its first statement on this subject in 1983, it continues to be controversial. There are those who believe that surrogacy should be permitted because such arrangements can be beneficial to all parties, and to prohibit them would limit the autonomy of infertile couples and surrogates. Others believe that the risks outweigh the benefits or that because of shifting emotions and attitudes toward the fetus during gestation, it is not possible for a pregnant woman to give truly informed consent to relinquish an infant until after birth has occurred (1).

Many issues related to surrogate motherhood have not been resolved, and considerable disagreement persists within the medical profession, the medical ethics community, state legislatures, the courts, and the general public. Similarly, no one position reflects the variety of opinions on surrogacy within ACOG's membership. While recognizing these differences of opinion, this chapter will focus on the ethical responsibilities of obstetrician–gynecologists who choose to participate in surrogacy arrangements on a variety of levels, including caring for the pregnant woman and her fetus.

The first part of the chapter provides an overview of public policy issues, descriptions of the types of surrogacy, arguments supporting and opposing surrogacy arrangements, and particular concerns related to payment and commercialization. The second part offers ethical recommendations to physicians who are involved in counseling infertile couples or potential surrogate mothers, who provide obstetric services for pregnant surrogates, or who offer assisted reproductive techniques using surrogacy. The ethical obligations of physicians will vary depending on the type and level of their involvement in surrogacy arrangements.

General Issues

Public Policy

In some states, the practice of surrogate motherhood is not clearly covered under existing law. There is a split among the states that have statutes. Some states prohibit surrogacy contracts or make them void and unenforceable, while others permit such agreements (2).

When a court is asked to decide a dispute regarding parental rights or custody of a child born as a result of a surrogacy arrangement, existing statutes may not prove adequate because of the complexity of the problem. Courts faced with such decisions have given preference to different factors: the best interest of the child, the rights of the birth mother (as in adoption situations), the genetic link between the child and the genetic parents, and the intent of the couple who entered into a surrogacy contract to become parents. Often 2 or more of these factors conflict with each other, and there is no consensus in the legal or ethical communities as to which should have priority (2–6).

The obstetrician–gynecologist who facilitates surrogacy arrangements should be aware of any statutes or court cases in the state in which he or she practices. In counseling individuals seeking a child through surrogacy or a woman who is considering becoming a surrogate, the physician should encourage them to consider the possible consequences of a surrogacy arrangement, including potential legal complications.

Previously published as Committee Opinion 225, November 1999

Types of Surrogacy

Surrogacy can be classified on the basis of the source of the genetic material. Eggs, sperm, or both may be donated, thereby altering the "intended parents'" biologic relationship to the child.

In one type of surrogacy arrangement, the intended parents are a couple who reach an agreement with a woman (the "surrogate mother") who will be artificially inseminated with sperm provided by the male partner of the couple seeking surrogacy services. Thus, the genetic and gestational mother of any resultant child is the surrogate mother, and the genetic father is the intended father. The intended parents plan to be the "social" or "rearing" parents of the child. Although this chapter refers to a couple as intended parents, individuals also may seek surrogacy services.

In another type of surrogacy, in vitro fertilization and embryo transfer are combined with surrogate parenting arrangements. In this case, it is possible for both the intended father and the intended mother to be the genetic parents of the child, and the surrogate fulfills only the role of gestational mother. This type of arrangement originally was called surrogate gestational motherhood, and now the carrying woman is called the "gestational carrier" or "gestational surrogate."

The different types of relationships that are possible—genetic (either, both, or neither intended parent), gestational (the surrogate), and social or rearing (the intended parents)—give rise to both conceptual problems about the nature of parenthood and legal problems as to who should be considered the parents responsible for the child.

Major Arguments for and Against Surrogate Parenthood Arrangements

Surrogate parenthood can allow a couple to have a child when they would otherwise be unable to do so except by adoption, because of an inability to achieve pregnancy or medical contraindications to pregnancy for the intended mother. Adoption, however, does not provide a genetic link to the child, an important consideration for some prospective parents. Surrogate parenthood is chosen by some prospective parents because of a desire for genetic linkage or for practical reasons, such as the scarcity of adoptable children.

Arguments based on reproductive liberty also support surrogate parenthood arrangements. In the United States, the freedom to decide whether and when to conceive or bear a child is a highly protected right. Thus, some have argued that intended parents and surrogate mothers should be free to cooperate in procreating, at least in cases of medical need and where care is taken to avoid harming others, especially the prospective child. Furthermore, the surrogate mother may derive satisfaction from helping the intended parents. Some women become surrogates primarily for altruistic reasons and see their services as a gift.

The primary arguments against surrogate motherhood are based on the harms that the practice may be thought to produce—harms to the child that is born, harms to the surrogate herself, harms to her existing children if she has children, and harms to society as a whole. It is surely harmful to any child to be the object of a custody dispute. In addition, the rejection of an infant—for example, rejection of a disabled infant by both intended parents and surrogate mother—is a significant harm. If an existing relationship is used to coerce relatives or close friends to become surrogate mothers, that coercion is a harm resulting from the practice of surrogate motherhood. The existing children of a surrogate mother may be harmed if her pregnancy and relinquishment result in high levels of stress for the surrogate or her family. These children and society as a whole may be harmed by the perception that reproduction is trivialized by transactions that translate women's reproductive capacities and the infants that result into commodities to be bought and sold. Depersonalization of a pregnant woman as a "vehicle" for the genetic perpetuation of other individuals may harm not only surrogate mothers but also the status of women as a whole. There also is a concern that redefining concepts of motherhood may threaten traditional understandings of parenting and family.

Children are much more vulnerable than adults. Harms to children who have no choice in a matter are more serious, from an ethical standpoint, than harms to adults who make a choice that they later regret. Further, a distinction should be drawn between harms that inevitably, or almost invariably, are associated with a practice and harms that perhaps could be avoided through advance planning, appropriate counseling, or oversight mechanisms.

Few studies provide data about harms and benefits resulting from surrogate parenting arrangements. Speculative discussion about possible outcomes does not provide a solid foundation for ethical conclusions and clinical guidelines. It is important to know whether these outcomes actually occur and, if so, how frequently. Studies that will provide more data of this type are needed (7, 8).

In summary, there are strong arguments both for and against the practice of surrogate parenthood. Physicians will be on both sides of this debate. If, after careful consideration of the arguments, a physician chooses to facilitate or recommend surrogacy arrangements, then all precautions should be taken to prevent medical, psychologic, and legal harms to the intended parents, the potential surrogate, and the prospective child.

Payment to the Surrogate Mother

Perhaps no topic related to surrogate motherhood is more contentious than compensation of the surrogate mother by the intended parents (9). Payment to surrogates often is substantial because of the duration and complexity of involvement. As noted previously, some states specifically prohibit surrogacy contracts that involve payment. Several questions about payment for surrogacy should be raised:

For what is payment made? Although there is debate on this point, it is clear that payment must not be made contingent on the delivery of an "acceptable product"—a live-born, healthy child. Rather, payment should be construed as compensation for the surrogate mother's time and effort, her initiating and carrying the pregnancy, her giving birth to an infant, her acceptance of the risks of pregnancy and childbirth, and her possible loss of employment opportunities.

Why is payment offered or requested? In many surrogate parenthood arrangements among close friends or relatives, there is no payment for the services of the surrogate. Rather, the surrogate may provide her services as an act of altruism, and the intended parents will be asked to reimburse her only for out-of-pocket expenses connected with the pregnancy. However, most women are understandably reluctant to undertake the burdens and risks of pregnancy on behalf of strangers without some kind of compensation for their time, effort, and risk.

Is payment likely to lead to the exploitation of potential surrogates? Surrogacy arrangements often take place between parties with unequal power, education, and economic status (10). Unless independent legal representation and mental health counseling are mandated, women serving as surrogates may be particularly vulnerable to being treated as commodities. If a payment offered to a candidate for surrogacy is too low, it may be said to exploit her by not providing adequate compensation; if the payment is too high, it may be said to exploit her by being irresistible and coercive. Opponents of surrogate moth-

erhood also have argued that if a fee must be paid to the surrogate mother, only affluent couples will be able to seek surrogacy services. This access barrier exists, however, for most services related to infertility, for certain other medical procedures, and for adoption, and thus is not specific to surrogacy agreements.

Responsibilities of Obstetrician–Gynecologists

Ethical recommendations in this chapter focus on 4 categories of physician involvement: 1) advising couples who are considering surrogacy, 2) counseling potential surrogate mothers, 3) providing obstetric services for pregnant surrogates, and 4) offering assisted reproductive techniques related to surrogacy. Although the obligations of physicians will vary depending on the type and level of their involvement, in all cases physicians should carefully examine all relevant issues, including medical, ethical, legal, and psychologic aspects.

Intended parents and surrogate mothers have both divergent and common interests. Because of these divergent interests, one professional individual (eg, physician, attorney, or psychologist) or agency should not represent the interests of both major parties in surrogate parenting arrangements. The physician who treats the intended parents should not have the surrogate mother as an obstetric patient, because conflicts of interest may arise that would not allow the physician to serve all parties properly.

Responsibilities of Physicians to Couples Considering Surrogacy

When approached by a couple considering surrogacy, the physician should, as in all other aspects of medical care, be certain that there will be a full discussion of ethical and legal issues as well as medical risks, benefits, and alternatives, many of which have been addressed in this statement. An obstetrician–gynecologist who is not familiar with these issues should refer the couple for appropriate counseling. Additional recommendations for advising couples considering surrogacy are as follows:

- Because of the risks inherent in surrogacy arrangements, such arrangements should be considered only in the case of infertility or health-related needs, not for convenience alone.
- A physician may justifiably decline to participate in initiating surrogate motherhood arrangements for personal, ethical, or medical reasons.

- If a physician decides to become involved in facilitating surrogate motherhood arrangements, the following guidelines should be used:

    — The physician should be assured that appropriate procedures are used to screen the intended parents and the surrogate. Such screening should include appropriate fertility studies, medical screening, and psychologic assessment.

    — Mental health counseling should be provided before initiation of a pregnancy 1) to permit the potential surrogate and the intended parents to explore the range of outcomes and possible long-term effects and 2) to consider possible psychologic risks to and vulnerabilities of both parties and the prospective child.

    — It is preferable that surrogate parenting arrangements be overseen by private nonprofit agencies with credentials similar to those of adoption agencies. However, many existing agencies are entrepreneurial and for-profit (8). A physician making a referral to an agency must have assurance that the agency is medically and ethically reputable and that it is committed to protecting the interests of all parties involved.

    — The physician should receive only usual compensation for medical services. Referral fees and other arrangements for financial gain beyond usual fees for medical services are inappropriate.

    — The physician should not refer patients to surrogacy programs in which the financial arrangements are likely to exploit any of the parties.

- The obstetrician–gynecologist should urge the intended parents to discuss preconditions and possible contingencies with the surrogate or her rep-resentative and to agree in advance on the response to them. These include, but may not be limited to, the expected health-related behaviors of the surrogate; the prenatal diagnosis of a genetic or chromosomal abnormality; the inability or unwillingness of the surrogate to carry the pregnancy to term; the death of one of the intended parents or the dissolution of the couple's marriage during the pregnancy; the birth of an infant with a disability; a decision by the surrogate mother to abrogate the contract and to contest custody of an infant conceived through the sperm of the intended father; or, in the case of gestational surrogacy, the option of registering the intended parents as the legal parents.

- The obstetrician–gynecologist should urge the parties involved to record in writing the preconditions and contingency plans on which they have agreed to make explicit the intentions of the parties, to facilitate later recollection of these intentions, and to help promote the interests of the future child. In the preparation of this agreement, both parties should be encouraged to have independent legal representation.

- Whatever compensation is provided to the surrogate mother should be paid solely on the basis of her time and effort, her initiating and carrying the pregnancy, her giving birth to an infant, her acceptance of the risks of pregnancy and childbirth, and her possible loss of employment opportunities. Compensation must not be contingent on a successful delivery or on the health of the child.

- Where possible, obstetrician–gynecologists should cooperate with and participate in research intended to provide data on outcomes of surrogacy arrangements.

Responsibilities of Physicians to Potential Surrogates

When approached by a patient considering becoming a surrogate mother, the physician should address ethical and legal concerns fully along with medical risks and benefits as part of the initial consultation. In particular, the physician should be sure that preconditions and contingencies, such as those outlined in the previous section, have been thoroughly considered and that the potential surrogate recognizes the importance of having explicit written precondition and contingency agreements. In the preparation of this agreement, both parties should be encouraged to have independent legal representation. Additional recommendations for counseling and providing other services for potential surrogate mothers are as follows:

- To avoid conflict of interest, the physician should not facilitate a woman's becoming a surrogate mother for a couple whom the physician also is treating.

- The physician should ensure that appropriate procedures are used to screen and counsel both the intended parents and the surrogate. Referral for mental health counseling should be provided before initiation of a pregnancy 1) to permit the potential surrogate to explore the range of outcomes and possible long-term effects and 2) to evaluate her psychologic risks and vulnerabilities as well as the possible effects of surrogacy on her existing relationships and on any existing children.

- A physician who provides examinations and performs procedures for an agency that arranges surrogacy contracts should be aware of the policies of the agency and should decline involvement with any agency whose policies are not consistent with the ethical recommendations of this chapter and those of other professional organizations related to reproductive medicine, such as the American Society for Reproductive Medicine (formerly known as the American Fertility Society) (7, 8).

- Whatever compensation is provided to the surrogate mother should be paid solely on the basis of her time and effort, her initiating and carrying the pregnancy, her giving birth to an infant, her acceptance of the risks of pregnancy and childbirth, and her possible loss of employment opportunities. Compensation must not be contingent on a successful delivery or on the health of the child.

- The physician should avoid participation in medical care arising from surrogacy arrangements in which the financial or other arrangements are likely to exploit any of the parties. The physician is therefore obliged to become as informed as possible about the financial and other arrangements between the surrogate and intended parents to make ethical decisions about providing medical care. A physician who agrees to provide medical care in what he or she assesses as clearly exploitative circumstances has a responsibility to discuss problematic arrangements with all parties and may choose to transfer care when it is possible to do so.

Responsibilities of Physicians to Pregnant Surrogates

When a pregnant surrogate seeks medical care for an established pregnancy, the obstetrician should explore with the surrogate her understanding of her contract with the intended parents and any provisions of it that may affect her care. If the physician believes that provisions of the contract may conflict with his or her professional judgment, the physician may refuse to accept the patient under those terms. Once accepted as a patient, she should be cared for as any other obstet-

ric patient, regardless of the method of conception, or referred to an obstetrician who will provide that care. Additional recommendations regarding the provision of obstetric services to surrogates are as follows:

- The obstetrician's professional obligation is to support the well-being of the pregnant woman and her fetus, to support the pregnant woman's goals for the pregnancy, and to provide appropriate care regardless of the patient's plans to keep or relinquish the future child. If a physician's discomfort with surrogacy arrangements might interfere with that obligation, the patient should be referred to another obstetrician.

- The pregnant surrogate should be the sole source of consent regarding clinical intervention and management of the pregnancy, labor, and delivery.

- Agreements the surrogate has made with the intended parents regarding her care and behavior during pregnancy and delivery should not affect the physician's care of the patient. The obstetrician must make recommendations that are in the best interests of the pregnant woman and her fetus, regardless of prior agreements between her and the intended parents.

- Confidentiality between the physician and the pregnant patient should be maintained. The intended parents may have access to the patient's medical information only with her explicit consent.

- Obstetrician–gynecologists are encouraged to assist in the development of hospital policies to address labor, delivery, postpartum, and neonatal care in situations in which surrogacy arrangements exist.

Responsibilities of Infertility Specialists and Reproductive Endocrinologists to Intended Parents and Surrogates

In providing medical services related to surrogate motherhood arrangements, infertility specialists and reproductive endocrinologists should follow the recommendations in the 2 previous sections. In particular, these specialists should ensure that appropriate procedures are used to screen the intended parents and the surrogate and that mental health counseling is provided to all parties before initiation of a pregnancy. Additional recommendations regarding the provision of assisted reproductive techniques are as follows:

- A physician who performs artificial insemination or in vitro fertilization as a part of surrogacy services necessarily will have to deal with both the intended parents and the surrogate. However, the couple and the surrogate should have independent counseling and independent legal representation, and the surrogate should obtain obstetric care from a physician who is not involved with the intended parents.
- A physician who provides examinations and performs procedures for an agency that arranges surrogacy contracts should be aware of the policies of the agency and should decline involvement with any agency whose policies are not consistent with the ethical recommendations of this chapter and those of other professional organizations related to reproductive medicine (7, 8).
- Specialists in infertility and reproductive endocrinology are encouraged to participate in research that is intended to provide data on the outcomes of surrogacy arrangements.

Summary

The obstetrician–gynecologist has an ethical responsibility to review the risks and benefits of surrogate parenthood fully and fairly with couples who are considering surrogacy arrangements. The obstetrician who is consulted by a pregnant woman who has made surrogacy arrangements owes her the same care as any pregnant woman and must respect her right to be the sole source of consent for all matters regarding prenatal care and delivery. The gynecologist or specialist in reproductive endocrinology who performs procedures required for surrogacy should be guided by the same ethical principles aimed at safeguarding the well-being of all participants, including the future child.

References

1. Lederman RP. Psychosocial adaptation in pregnancy: assessment of seven dimensions of maternal development. New York (NY): Springer Publishing Company; 1996.
2. The American Surrogacy Center, Inc. Legal overview of surrogacy laws by state. Marietta (GA): TASC; 1997. Available at http://www.surrogacy.com/legals/map.html. Retrieved July 29, 2003.
3. Andrews LB. Alternative modes of reproduction. In: Cohen S, Taub N, editors. Reproductive laws for the 1990s. Clifton (NJ): Humana Press; 1989. p. 361–403.
4. Serratelli A. Surrogate motherhood contracts: should the British or Canadian model fill the U.S. legislative vacuum? George Washington J Int Law Econ 1993;26:633–74.
5. Field M. Reproductive technologies and surrogacy: legal issues. Creighton Law Rev 1992;25:1589–98.
6. New York State Task Force on Life and the Law. Assisted reproductive technologies: analysis and recommendations for public policy. New York (NY): NYSTF; 1998.
7. Surrogate gestational mothers: women who gestate a genetically unrelated embryo. American Fertility Society. Fertil Steril 1994;62 (5 suppl):67S–70S.
8. Surrogate mothers. American Fertility Society. Fertil Steril 1994;62 (5 suppl):71S–7S.
9. Moody-Adams MM. On surrogacy: morality, markets, and motherhood. Public Aff Q 1991;5:175–90.
10. Harrison M. Financial incentives for surrogacy. Womens Health Issues 1991;1:145–7.

Suggested Reading

National Conference of Commissioners on Uniform State Laws. Gestational agreement. Article 8. In: Uniform parentage act. Chicago (IL): NCCUSL; 2002. p. 68–78.

Sterilization of Women, Including Those With Mental Disabilities

Sterilization, like any other surgical procedure, must be carried out under the general ethical principles of patient autonomy and beneficence. Special ethical considerations are imposed by the unique attributes of sterilization. The procedure usually is done not for medical indications, but electively for family planning. It may have a significant impact on individuals other than the patient, especially her partner. It is intended to be permanent, although techniques are available to attempt reversal or circumvention of sterility. Finally, sterilization affects procreation and, therefore, may conflict with the moral beliefs of the patient, her family, or the physician. When the patient has diminished mental abilities or chronic mental illness, even more stringent ethical constraints apply.

General Ethical Principles

Under the principle of autonomy, patients have the right to seek, accept, or refuse care. Sterilization is for many a social choice rather than purely a medical issue, but all patient-related activities engaged in by physicians are subject to the same ethical guidelines. Patients sometimes request a physician's counsel in deciding whether to request sterilization. Physicians should be cautious in giving advice and making recommendations that go beyond health-related issues, even though nonmedical factors might be the most compelling for the patient. It may be difficult for the physician to address nonmedical issues without bias. Also, the physician may not have a full understanding of the patient's situation. However, it is entirely appropriate for the physician to assist the patient in exploring and articulating the reasons for her decision.

Previously published as Committee Opinion 216, April 1999; content revised January 2004

Although a woman's request for sterilization may conflict with the physician's medical judgment or moral beliefs, the patient's values must be respected. In such cases, the physician has an obligation to inform the patient of his or her professional recommendation and the medical reasons for it. The physician remains responsible for his or her actions and is not obligated to act in violation of personal principles of conscience, but the patient should be informed of such principles if she inquires. If the patient continues to desire sterilization, the physician has the obligation to refer her to another caregiver or at least to inform her that sterilization services may be available elsewhere. The physician's values, sense of societal goals, and racial, ethnic, or socioeconomic issues should not be the basis of a recommendation to undergo sterilization.

Sterilization requires the patient's informed consent for ethical and medical–legal reasons. The physician performing the procedure has the responsibility of ensuring that the patient is properly counseled concerning the risks and benefits of sterilization. The patient should receive comprehensive and individualized counseling on reversible alternatives to sterilization (1). The procedure's intended permanence should be stressed, as well as the possibility of future regret. An estimate of the procedure's failure rate and risk of ectopic pregnancy should be provided. A variety of patient education materials are available to assist in preoperative counseling, but it is essential for the patient to be given the opportunity to discuss all relevant issues with her physician and to ask questions.

The physician should be familiar with any laws and regulations that may constrain sterilization, such as limitations on the patient's age and requirements for the consent process. The physician should inform the patient that insurance coverage for sterilization is variable so that she can discuss this issue with her insurer.

Specific Ethical Issues

Because sterilization may have important effects on individuals other than the patient, women requesting sterilization should be encouraged to discuss the issues with their families, especially their sexual partners. In many cases, it is preferable for the male partner to be sterilized. It may be helpful for the physician to counsel the partner directly, with the patient's consent.

Hysterectomy solely for the purpose of sterilization is inappropriate. The risks and cost of the procedure are disproportionate to the benefit, given the available alternatives. In disabled women with limited functional capability, indications for major surgical procedures remain the same as in other patients. In all cases, indications for surgery must meet standard criteria, and the benefits of the procedure must exceed known procedural risks. Disabled women with limited functional capacity may sometimes be physically unable to care for their menstrual hygiene and are profoundly disturbed by their menses. On occasion, such women's caretakers have sought hysterectomy for these indications. Hysterectomy for the purpose of cessation of normal menses may be considered after other reasonable alternatives have been attempted.

Women may be vulnerable to various forms of coercion in their medical decision making. For example, the withholding of other medical care by linking it to the patient's consent to undergo sterilization is ethically unacceptable. Laws, regulations, and reimbursement restrictions concerning sterilization have been created to protect vulnerable individuals, including those with mental disabilities, from abuse. However, sterilization should not be denied to individuals simply because they also may be vulnerable to coercion. Physicians caring for patients who request or require procedures that result in sterilization may find themselves in a dilemma when legal and reimbursement restrictions interfere with a patient's choice of treatment. Rigid timing and age requirements can restrict access to good health care and result in unnecessary risk (2). Physicians are encouraged to seek legal or ethical consultation or both whenever necessary in their efforts to provide care that is most appropriate in individual situations.

At a public policy level, the medical profession has an opportunity to be a voice of reason and compassion by pointing out when legislative and regulatory measures intended to be safeguards interfere with patient choice and appropriate medical care.

Special Considerations Concerning Patients With Mental Disabilities

As used in this chapter, the term "women with mental disabilities" refers to individuals whose ability to participate in the informed consent process is, or might be, limited and whose autonomy is, or might be, thereby impaired. Such individuals constitute a heterogeneous group, including those with varying degrees of presumably irreversible "mental retardation," as well as those with varying types and degrees of "chronic mental illness." Some of these illnesses are reversible to varying degrees and for varying periods. The concept of "chronically and variably impaired autonomy" has been proposed to describe such situations (3).

Physicians who perform sterilizations must be aware of widely differing federal, state, and local laws and regulations, which have arisen in reaction to a long and unhappy history of sterilization of "unfit" individuals in the United States and elsewhere. The potential remains for serious abuses and injustices. Individuals who are capable of reproducing and parenting without a presumptive risk of child neglect or abuse may be deprived of their procreative rights simply because they carry a label such as mild retardation that suggests an inherent unfitness to parent. The implications of this labeling process for reproductive rights should be examined as thoroughly and objectively as possible before arriving at a decision about sterilization.

Conversely, individuals for whom pregnancy is a serious burden or harm may be denied the opportunity for a full range of contraceptive options. For example, federal funds may not be used for the sterilization of "mentally incompetent" or "institutionalized" individuals (2). Physicians should always have the maximum respect for patient autonomy, and the presence of a mental disability does not, in itself, justify either sterilization or its denial.

Determination of Ability To Give Informed Consent

Before carrying out any surgical procedure, the physician has the important responsibility of ascertaining the patient's capacity to provide informed consent. It may be difficult to be sure that patients with normal intellectual function understand the complexities of some situations; when the patient has a mental disability, the task is more difficult and the responsibility is more challenging.

Evaluating a mentally impaired patient's ability to provide informed consent is seldom straightforward (4). For example, although degrees of mental retardation have been defined according to intelligence quotient, there is no direct relationship between such diagnostic categories and the capacity to consent. Among the issues that may need to be considered in the assessment are the patient's language and culture, the quality of information provided (clarity, completeness, lack of bias), the setting of counseling (privacy, comfort), and possible fluctuations in the patient's comprehension. Such fluctuations may result from various stressors and medications. Multiple interviews over an adequate period may be required. Obtaining the assistance of professionals trained in communicating with mentally disabled individuals is essential. These professionals may include special educators, psychologists, nurses, attorneys familiar with disability law, and physicians accustomed to working with mentally disabled patients.

The process of evaluating a patient's ability to give informed consent may be set forth in laws of the jurisdiction involved, and legal requirements for the determination of competence vary greatly. The concept of legal competence is quite complex. Standards for the definition of competence may vary with the specific purpose (eg, marriage, making a will, consenting or refusing life-saving treatment, or, as in the case of sterilization, consenting to elective surgery).

Court approval of sterilization may be required by law or may be necessary in difficult cases because of disagreement among the patient's caregivers and consultants. In most jurisdictions, court action is not required to carry out a sterilization procedure if there is agreement among these consultants that a nonminor is capable of consenting. Certain jurisdictions may not recognize guardian consent for sterilization of minors with mental disabilities under any circumstances. Whether or not recourse to the courts is necessary, every effort should be made to conduct the determination of competence fairly and to preserve autonomy.

Ethical Issues When the Patient Cannot Give Informed Consent

When the patient has been determined to be irreversibly incapable of participating in all or part of the informed consent process, others must make beneficence-based decisions regarding medical treatment. Such a determination is relatively uncommon. Even in these situations, it often is possible and highly desirable to obtain at least the patient's assent. The initial premise should be that nonvoluntary sterilization generally is not ethically acceptable because of the violation of privacy, bodily integrity, and reproductive rights that it may represent.

Physicians and other caregivers should avoid paternalistic decisions in all cases in which the individual may be capable of participating to some degree in decisions regarding her care. The following recommendations are based in part on those of McCullough et al (3). They do not apply to mentally impaired individuals who can participate in the consent process.

For patients with chronically and variably impaired autonomy, initial efforts should be directed toward restoring decision-making ability by such means as adjustment of medication and avoidance of stressors. This may allow the patient to exercise full autonomy. For cases in which these efforts fail, the following guidelines are recommended:

- Efforts should be made to conform to the patient's expressed values and beliefs regarding reproduction. Such information may be available from interviewing the patient, her family, caregivers, and others in her environment. If possible, alternatives (including no action) consistent with her beliefs, medical condition, and social situation should be presented to decision makers.

- Physicians should be aware of the possibility of undue pressure from family members whose interests, no matter how legitimate, may not be the same as the patient's. When appropriate, the patient should have the opportunity to be interviewed without family members present.

- Noninvasive modalities designed to assist family members and other caregivers with setting behavioral limits should be considered as alternatives to sterilization. These resources may include socialization training, sexual abuse avoidance training, supportive family therapy, and sexuality education.

- Consideration should be given to the degree of certainty of various adverse outcomes. For example, given the patient's living circumstances, how likely is it that she might be sexually exploited? Given available knowledge concerning her reproductive potential (ovulatory status, tubal patency), how likely is it that she will become pregnant? How likely are adverse medical or social consequences from a pregnancy? Because it is uncommon for such risks to be reliably predictable, it may be preferable to recommend a reversible long-term form of contraception, such as an intrauterine device, long-term injectable progestin, or long-acting subdermal progestin implants (when available in the United States), instead of sterilization. In most cases, the chosen method of contraception should be the least restrictive in preserving future reproductive options. This is especially true when a major factor in the request for sterilization is concern about burdens for others. At the same time, risks and inconveniences of contraception over a long period, as compared with a single, relatively simple and definitive surgical procedure, should not be ignored.

- The well-being of a child potentially conceived also should receive consideration.

Summary

Sterilization is an elective procedure with permanent and far-reaching consequences. Physicians who perform sterilization have ethical responsibilities of the highest order to counsel patients fully and without bias. Physicians must assess thoroughly the capacity of patients with impaired mental abilities to participate fully in the informed consent process. When this capacity is limited, the physician must consult with the patient's other caregivers in reaching a decision, which is based on the patient's best interests and preserves her autonomy to the maximum extent possible. In difficult cases, a hospital ethics committee may provide useful perspectives.

References

1. Benefits and risks of sterilization. ACOG Practice Bulletin No. 46. American College of Obstetricians and Gynecologists. Obstet Gynecol 2003;102:647–58.
2. Sterilization of persons in federally assisted family planning projects. 42 C.F.R. § 50 Subpart B (2002).
3. McCullough LB, Coverdale J, Bayer T, Chervenak FA. Ethically justified guidelines for family planning interventions to prevent pregnancy in female patients with chronic mental illness. Am J Obstet Gynecol 1992;167:19–25.
4. Appelbaum PS, Grisso T. Assessing patients' capacities to consent to treatment [published erratum appears in N Engl J Med 1989;320:748]. N Engl J Med 1988;319:1635–8.

End-of-Life Decision Making

The expressions "withdrawal and withholding of treatment" and "treatment refusal" are reflective of an ethos that has shaped American medical research and practice for the last half century. That ethos regards the use of interventionist strategies to promote cure and prolong life as the physician's primary obligation. Consequently, any decision not to embrace such strategies has been construed negatively as a "withholding," a "withdrawal," or a "refusal." The purpose of this chapter is to encourage a move away from these terms and the assumptions that they embody about the aims of caregiving. It suggests a more open, collaborative approach to clinical decision making, one grounded in the explicit identification of the operative goals of care. In particular, this chapter emphasizes the dignity, appropriateness, and ethical probity of palliation and comfort as caregiving goals. The 18th century was another era in which the duty to cure and prolong life was regarded as paramount by physicians. Medical essayist John Gregory's 1772 exhortation to his colleagues continues to be germane in this regard: "It is as much the business of a physician…to alleviate pain, and to smooth the avenues of death as to cure diseases" (1).

This chapter discusses the process of communication that leads to the identification of the goals of care and, in particular, to the goals that may direct end-of-life caregiving in obstetrics and gynecology. As a foundation for this discussion, this chapter addresses 1) the ethical values that undergird medical practice, and 2) the legal developments that bear on end-of-life decision making.

The Ethical Basis of Medical Practice

The moral character of medicine is based on 3 values central to the healing relationship. They are

Previously published as Committee Opinion 156, May 1995; content revised January 2004

patient benefit, patient self-determination, and the ethical integrity of the health care professional (2, 3).

Patient Benefit

The obligation to promote the good of the patient is a basic presumption of medical caregiving and a defining feature of the physician's ethical responsibility. To promote the patient's good is to provide care in which benefits outweigh burdens or harms. Benefits, in turn, are understood only relative to the goals that the patient and physician hope to achieve through medical care.

Patient Self-Determination

The inherent value of individual autonomy or self-determination is one of the fundamental bases of democracy and of individual rights and protections in the United States. In health care, the value of individual autonomy is affirmed in the ethical and legal doctrine of informed consent (see "Informed Consent" in Part I) (4). Under this doctrine, the patient has a right to control what happens to her body. This means that no treatment may be given to the patient without her consent (or, if she lacks decision-making capacity, the consent of her valid surrogate). This right is not contingent on the presence or absence of terminal illness, on the agreement of family members, or on the approval of physicians or hospital administrators.

In the medical context, physician respect for patient self-determination consists of an active inclusion of the patient in decisions regarding her own care. This involves frank discussion of diagnoses and prognoses, the relative risks and benefits of alternative (including no) treatments, and, based on these discussions, a mutual identification of the operative goals of care. There is a strong presumption that all information needed to make health care decisions be provided to patients (or to their surrogates). Studies suggest that most patients want to know the reality of their conditions and benefit from an honest communication with the physician (5, 6). It is unethical for a physician to deny patients important information to avoid physician–patient interactions that are difficult or uncomfortable. Moreover, appropriate regard for patient autonomy involves respecting the patient's considered choice to change therapeutic modalities to better meet her current goals of care.

The Ethical Integrity of the Health Care Professional

Because physicians, like patients, are autonomous agents, they cannot be compelled to violate personal ethical or religious commitments in the service of the patient's good. If physicians have moral reservations about certain forms of caregiving, they should make that known at the outset. Although physicians are not obliged to do things that are at odds with their conscience, they must not stand in the way of patients' desires to seek other caregivers and should, where possible, help guide the transition.

The profession of medicine is guided by its moral commitment to avoid risks to the patient that are greater than potential benefits. On this basis, physicians have a presumptive obligation not to provide treatments that are untested, contraindicated, or useless. For this reason, a patient's demand for care that she deems desirable is not sufficient to impose on providers an absolute obligation to provide that care.

Legal Developments That Bear on End-of-Life Decision Making

In the 1990s, there were a number of developments in the law that bear on end-of-life decision making. First, in June 1990, in a decision on the Cruzan case, the United States Supreme Court affirmed that patients have a constitutionally protected right to refuse unwanted medical treatments (7). The ruling reaffirms states' authority to adopt procedural requirements for the withdrawal and withholding of life-prolonging medical interventions.

A second legal development was the passage of the federal Patient Self-Determination Act (PSDA), which went into effect December 1, 1991 (8). The PSDA requires Medicaid- and Medicare-participating health care institutions to inform all adult patients of their rights "to make decisions concerning medical care, including the right to accept or refuse medical or surgical treatment and the right to formulate an advance directive." Under the PSDA, institutions are legally required to provide this information to patients on admission for care or on enrollment in a health maintenance organization. The institution must note in the medical record the existence of an advance directive and must respect these directives to the fullest extent under state law. Put simply, the aim of the PSDA is to empower patients to make decisions regarding their medical care.

An advance directive is the formal mechanism by which a patient may express her values regarding her future health status. It may take the form of a proxy directive or an instructional directive or both. Proxy directives, such as the durable power of attorney for health care, designate a surrogate to make medical decisions on behalf of the patient who is no longer competent to express her choices. Instructional directives, such as "living wills," focus on the types of life-sustaining treatment that a patient would or would not choose in various clinical circumstances.

A third related development is found in limitations on the autonomy of the pregnant woman in the area of treatment refusal. Although courts at times have intervened, currently there is general agreement that a pregnant woman who has decision-making capacity has the same right to refuse treatment as a nonpregnant woman. Only in very exceptional circumstances would it be justifiable, either ethically or legally, to override this right (see "Patient Choice in the Maternal–Fetal Relationship" in Part II).

In the case of a pregnant woman who has lost decision-making capacity, either temporarily or permanently, the legal status is not as clear. In the situation of pregnancy, even a clear and explicit advance directive may not assure the woman that her treatment wishes will be followed (9). As of 2002, 31 states had living will statutes that explicitly forbid the withholding or withdrawal of life support either from all pregnant patients or from pregnant patients whose fetuses could become, or currently are, viable. Only 4 states specifically permit a woman to choose to refuse life-sustaining treatment if she is pregnant. The other states either have no living will statute or make no mention of pregnancy. Similar types of restrictions exist in some states with respect to a surrogate, proxy, or health care agent who is appointed to make decisions on behalf of a pregnant woman (10, 11) (see also "Patient Choice in the Maternal–Fetal Relationship" in Part II).

Statutes that prohibit pregnant women from exercising their right to choose or refuse medical treatment are ethically suspect and are likely to be challenged as unconstitutional. Women should not lose their rights when they become pregnant or terminally ill (12). Obstetrician–gynecologists should attempt to ensure that the wishes of their pregnant patients are followed. Even if the patient is no longer able to make her own decisions, her previously expressed wishes and values (whether expressed as an advance directive or through the appointment of a surrogate decision maker) should guide the course of treatment, whenever legally possible.

Physician–Patient Communication and the Goals of Care

The practice of obstetrics and gynecology involves many different types of caregiving. These include but are not limited to preventive care; periodic examinations; family planning; the provision of prenatal and delivery care; medical and surgical intervention for conditions that threaten a patient's fertility, life, or quality of life; long-term care for patients with chronic illness; and palliative care for patients whose illnesses offer no chance of cure or remission. Each of these types of caregiving is linked to definable goals that not only suggest the appropriate intensity and duration of care but also entail certain treatment modalities and rule out others. Questions about the use of specific therapeutic modalities become meaningful only in relation to the goals of management for a particular patient (13). Goals of care in obstetrics and gynecology include:

- Relief of symptoms, pain, and suffering
- Achievement of cure or remission
- Achievement or prevention of pregnancy
- Optimization of pregnancy outcomes
- Prevention of illness in a woman or her fetus or both
- Maintenance or restoration of biologic function
- Maximization of comfort
- Education of the patient about her medical condition

The operative goal or goals of care are properly identified through a process of shared and ongoing communication and decision making between the patient and physician (14–16). The physician also is responsible for initiating and coordinating communication with other members of the health care team so that decision making reflects the patient's entire medical condition and her identified goals of care. Explicit discussion about the goals of care is important for a number of reasons. First, assumptions about the objectives of care inevitably shape perceptions about the appropriate course of treatment. Second, these objectives may be understood differently by the patient and her caregivers. Third, unarticulated commitments to certain goals may lead to misunderstanding and conflict. Finally, the goals of care may evolve and change in response to clinical or other factors. A comprehensive and ongoing process of communication not only advances patient self-determination but also is the basis for "preventive ethics"; that is, the establishment of a moral common ground that may prevent ethical conflict and crisis (17).

Shared Decision Making Regarding the End of Life

The process of decision making regarding the end of life may take place under 2 different circumstances. In the first, decisions are made in a situation of present health crisis; these are immediate choices that determine actual end-of-life treatment. In the second, decisions are made that provide for possible future end-of-life situations; these decisions are expressed through advance directives.

Communication Regarding Immediate Health Status

An ongoing process of informed consent requires that physicians communicate information regarding the patient's health status and comparative risks and benefits of treatment (including no treatment) so that she or, if she lacks decision-making capacity, her surrogate may determine management goals. If the patient decides that the maximization of comfort is her desired goal of care, the practitioner's responsibilities will focus on palliative strategies, such as pain relief, attentive and responsive communication with the patient about her health status, and the facilitation of communication with the patient's involved family and loved ones. These components of care are essential to the physician's positive therapeutic role. For the general obstetrician–gynecologist whose patient is or has been under the care of a specialist physician, these often are the most valuable services that can be offered. The expression "nothing more can be done" is a misleading shorthand that improperly equates care with cure and, in so doing, ignores the importance of the physician's role in providing comfort to the dying patient (18–20).

In the face of end-of-life decision making, physicians trained to prize interventionist strategies must be especially careful not to impose their own conception of benefit or burden on a patient or to use coercive means to establish or achieve goals that are not shared by the patient. The obstetrician–gynecologist should recognize that the harms associated with prolonged attempts at cure may not be acceptable to the dying patient. However, neither the presence of a "Do Not Attempt Resuscitation" order nor specific directives regarding limitation of other treatments remove the responsibility for providing palliative care. Moreover, the physician should not rely on the presence or absence of a do not attempt resuscitation order to make assumptions about the appropriateness of other treatment but rather should be guided by the explicitly identified goals of care.

There is considerable evidence that sociocultural and gender differences between patients and their physicians may subtly influence the style and content of physician–patient communication and the care that patients receive (21–28). Physicians who are aware of these potential problems can guard against the influence of bias in judgments concerning patient choices. Differences in gender and in ethnic, social, religious, and economic background may complicate communication, but they should not compromise care.

If the patient or surrogate and physician finally disagree on the goals that should guide care, a clearly defined process of discussion and consultation should be followed to resolve the disagreement (see "Medical Futility" in Part II for an example of a process). By using such consultation to clarify the cultural, religious, or personal considerations that shape their decision making, the parties may be able to resolve apparent conflict.

Some patients who are near the end of life and who anticipate ever-increasing pain and suffering may inquire about the alternative of physician-assisted suicide. It currently is not legal for physicians to participate in physician-assisted suicide in states other than Oregon. When a patient inquires about physician-assisted suicide as a possible option, the physician should explore with her the nature of her fears and her expectations and should be prepared to offer reassurances regarding palliative care plans for relieving distress at the end of life. Physicians should be aware that a request for physician-assisted suicide, especially when the patient's current level of discomfort does not appear to be concordant with such a request, may be a marker for treatable depression.

Communication Regarding Future Health Status: The Advance Directive

The obstetrician–gynecologist often provides the primary access that women have to the health care system. In many cases, it is the obstetrician–gynecologist who not only acts as the principal physician for female patients but also has the most contact with them. For these reasons, the obstetrician–gynecologist is in an ideal position to discuss with the patient her values and wishes regarding future care and to encourage her to formulate an advance directive. As an expression of the patient's values regarding care, the advance directive is not qualitatively different from a patient's articulation of general and more immediate health care decisions. As such, discussion of the advance directive should be regarded as integral to the ongoing process of communication to be initiated by the health care provider (29–30).

A good opportunity to initiate the discussion of caregiving goals, including end-of-life care, is during well-patient care, either at the time of the periodic examination or during pregnancy. Because a patient's wishes regarding care might change over time or under different conditions of illness, these discussions should include occasional reexamination of values and goals and, if necessary, updating of the advance directive and other documentation. In other words, decision making should be treated as a process rather than an event (see "Informed Consent" in Part I).

To facilitate the initiation of these discussions, the patient history form could contain questions about a patient's execution of an advance directive and her designation of a surrogate or next of kin as her medical proxy. If the patient has an instructional directive or durable power of attorney or both, they should become part of her medical record. If the patient does not have an advance directive, assistance in executing one might be provided by the social services or nursing staff of a hospital or clinical practice.

Physician–patient communication regarding advance directives should first include information on the advance directive itself: the forms it may take and its purpose as an expression of the patient's rights in the direction of her own care. Second, the physician and patient should discuss the different goals that may now guide care and those that may come into play in the case of terminal illness. It should be made clear to the patient the types of therapy that could be used to advance these different goals. Third, where applicable, the physician and the patient should discuss possible scenarios where the patient's own prognosis and care might adversely affect the health of her fetus. Finally, the physician should discuss with the patient the importance of consistency between her written directive and the preferences she expresses to her health care proxy or next of kin or both. In the event that a patient loses the capacity for decision making, her interests can best be served if there is as much clarity and consistency as possible regarding her wishes.

Ideally, these discussions serve an educational purpose for both patient and physician. For the physician, these discussions establish a basis for future caregiving and provide an opportunity for the candid expression of personal values regarding care. For the patient, the discussions provide the opportunity to learn about advance directives, to formulate and articulate her values regarding the goals of care, and to understand the compatibility of these goals with the values of the provider.

Although it is the physician's responsibility to educate patients about possible future health status and rights regarding medical care, it is the responsibility of the patient to thoughtfully assess her values and goals and to make them clearly known to those involved in her care. Again, the explicit discussion of caregiving goals provides an optimal mechanism for shared decision making.

Surrogate Decision Making

If the patient who lacks decision-making capacity has not designated a health care proxy, state law may dictate the order in which relatives should be asked to serve as surrogates. The individual selected should be someone who knows the patient's values and wishes and will respect them in his or her role as surrogate decision maker. If there is conflict regarding the designation of a surrogate, it may be appropriate to seek the advice of an ethics committee or consultant or, possibly, the courts.

The surrogate decision maker is ethically obligated to base decisions on the wishes and values of the patient. If these wishes and values have been explicitly stated, either in writing or in oral discussion, the surrogate has to interpret and apply them in the current situation. If wishes and values have not been explicitly stated beforehand, the surrogate has to attempt to extrapolate them from what is known about the patient. In some cases, for example, a never-competent patient, the surrogate will have to rely entirely on an assessment as to what is in the best interests of this particular patient.

In proxy decision making for the dying patient, surrogates and health care providers should be aware that there is documentation of gender disparity in clinical medicine and research and in court decisions surrounding the right to refuse life-sustaining treatment. In a review of "right to die" cases, it was found that courts honored the previously stated treatment decisions of men in 75% of cases, whereas they respected the prior choices of female patients in only 14% of cases (31). Given the persistence and pervasiveness of social attitudes that take women's moral choices less seriously than men's, obstetrician–gynecologists and patient surrogates must prevent these biases from undermining their care of and advocacy for female patients. Likewise, this evidence should further motivate women to make their treatment decisions as explicit as possible in advance.

Pregnant Patients and End-of-Life Decisions: Preventing Conflict

For the overwhelming majority of pregnant women, the welfare of the fetus is of the utmost concern. This concern motivates women to modify their behaviors for months at a time and to undergo the discomforts and risks of pregnancy and delivery. This maternal interest in fetal welfare has traditionally been the basis of the fundamental ethical commitment of obstetrician–gynecologists: that they are responsible for both the pregnant woman and her fetus and that they must optimize the benefits to both while minimizing the risks to each.

Within the context of obstetric care, situations may arise when a dying pregnant woman must decide between caregiving goals that emphasize palliative management for her own illness or an interventionist strategy, such as cesarean delivery, for the sake of her fetus. Likewise, she might be forced to decide between a curative strategy, such as chemotherapy, for her metastatic breast cancer and a course that poses less risk to her fetus but offers her less anticipated benefit. In either case, it is safe to assume that having been provided with all of the clinical information necessary to make her decision, she regards the choice as a difficult, possibly excruciating one and one that she wishes she did not have to make. Because the patient with a life-threatening condition identifies treatment goals by weighing obligations and concerns for her family, her fetus, and her own health and life prospects, any decision that she makes is bound to jeopardize some of the things that she cares about.

To make these decisions, the pregnant patient will first and foremost need the best clinical information available on the relative risks and benefits of different management strategies for her and her fetus. Different views on the moral status of the fetus generate different positions regarding the fetus as a patient and, by extension, different positions regarding the physician's obligations to the fetus. When, because of divergent beliefs on this matter, risks and benefits are valued differently by patient and physician, there is a potential for conflict. This potential highlights the importance of candid discussion of these matters in advance of a situation of conflict or crisis. The proper course for resolving conflicts that do arise is discussion of the case with an ethics committee or consultant (see "Patient Choice in the Maternal–Fetal Relationship" in Part II) (17).

In the case of a pregnant patient who has lost decision-making capacity, current legal restrictions on advance directives and proxy decision makers may make it difficult to know and to consider the patient's treatment choices. As noted previously, obstetrician–gynecologists should anticipate such problems by prior discussion when possible and should use whatever mechanisms are legally available for respecting the woman's wishes regarding treatment (12).

Conclusion

Effective communication between the patient and the physician is the cornerstone of the therapeutic relationship. It provides the patient with the information she needs to make her health care decisions and it provides a common ground for the physician, the patient, her family, and other members of the health care team.

Questions about the use of specific therapeutic modalities become meaningful only in relation to the goals of management for the particular patient. Explicit identification of the operative goals of care is important, therefore, for 4 reasons: 1) assumptions about the objectives of care inevitably shape perceptions about the appropriate course of treatment; 2) these objectives may be understood differently by the patient and her caregivers; 3) unarticulated commitments to certain goals may lead to misunderstanding and conflict; and 4) the goals of care may evolve and change in response to clinical or other factors.

In the course of providing comprehensive care, obstetrician–gynecologists are in an ideal position to encourage women to formulate advance directives. As an expression of the patient's values regarding care, the advance directive is not qualitatively different from a patient's articulation of general and more immediate health care decisions. As such, discussion of the advance directive should be regarded as integral to the ongoing process of communication to be initiated by the health care provider. Special attention should be given to the discussion of treatment wishes with pregnant women, especially in view of current state restrictions on the application of advance directives during pregnancy.

Sometimes the maximization of comfort is the chosen therapeutic goal. In this case, the physician can continue to benefit the patient in a number of important ways by providing humane and supportive care at the end of life.

References

1. Pernick MS. The calculus of suffering in nineteenth-century surgery. Hastings Cent Rep 1983;13(2):26–36.
2. Pellegrino ED, Thomasma DC. For the patient's good: the restoration of beneficence in health care. New York (NY): Oxford University Press; 1988.
3. Beauchamp TL, Childress JF. Principles of biomedical ethics. 5th ed. New York (NY): Oxford University Press; 2001.
4. Faden RR, Beauchamp TL, King NM. A history and theory of informed consent. New York (NY): Oxford University Press; 1986.
5. Edinger W, Smucker DR. Outpatients' attitudes regarding advance directives. J Fam Pract 1992;35:650–3.
6. American Academy of Pediatrics Committee on Bioethics. Guidelines on foregoing life-sustaining medical treatment. Pediatrics 1994;93:532–6.
7. Cruzan v Director of the Missouri Dept. of Health et al, 497 US 261, 262 (1990).
8. Cate FH, Gill BA. The Patient Self-Determination Act: implementation issues and opportunities. Washington, DC: The Annenberg Washington Program; 1991.
9. Partnership for Caring. Women and end-of-life decisions. Washington, DC: PFC; 2001. Available at http://www.partnershipforcaring.org/Resources/women&eol02.html. Retrieved August 1, 2003.
10. Partnership for Caring. Pregnancy restrictions in living will statutes. March 2002. (800-989-9455).
11. Partnership for Caring. Pregnancy restrictions in statutes authorizing health care agents. March 2002. (800-989-9455).
12. Grodin MA. Women's health and end-of-life decision making. Womens Health Issues 1996;6:295–301.
13. American Medical Association, The Robert Wood Johnson Foundation. EPEC: education for physicians on end-of-life care: participant's handbook. Chicago (IL): AMA; Princeton (NJ): RWJF; 1999.
14. Larson DG, Tobin DR. End-of-life conversations: evolving practice and theory. JAMA 2000;284:1573–8.
15. Tulsky JA, Chesney MA, Lo B. How do medical residents discuss resuscitation with patients? J Gen Intern Med 1995;10:436–42.
16. Tulsky JA, Chesney MA, Lo B. See one, do one, teach one? House staff experience discussing do-not-resuscitate orders. Arch Intern Med 1996;156:1285–9.
17. McCullough LB, Chervenak FA. Ethics in obstetrics and gynecology. New York (NY): Oxford University Press; 1994.

18. Brody H, Campbell ML, Faber-Langendoen K, Ogle KS. Withdrawing intensive life-sustaining treatment—recommendations for compassionate clinical management. N Engl J Med 1997;336:652–7.

19. Faber-Langendoen K, Lanken PN. Dying patients in the intensive care unit: forgoing treatment, maintaining care. Ann Intern Med 2000;133:886–93.

20. Field MJ, Cassel CK, editors. Approaching death: improving care at the end of life. Washington, DC: National Academy Press; 1997.

21. Waitzkin H. Doctor-patient communication. Clinical implications of social scientific research. JAMA 1984; 252:2441–6.

22. Levy DR. White doctors and black patients: influence of race on the doctor–patient relationship. Pediatrics 1985; 75:639–43.

23. Kolder VE, Gallagher J, Parsons MT. Court-ordered obstetrical interventions. N Engl J Med 1987;316:1192–6.

24. Chasnoff IJ, Landress HJ, Barrett ME. The prevalence of illicit-drug or alcohol use during pregnancy and discrepancies in mandatory reporting in Pinellas County, Florida. N Engl J Med 1990;322:1202–6.

25. Roter D, Lipkin M Jr, Korsgaard A. Sex differences in patients' and physicians' communication during primary care medical visits. Med Care 1991;29:1083–93.

26. Lurie N, Slater J, McGovern P, Ekstrum J, Quam L, Margolis K. Preventive care for women. Does the sex of the physician matter? N Engl J Med 1993;329:478–82.

27. Farley MA. North American bioethics: a feminist critique. In: Grodin MA, editor. Meta medical ethics: the philosophical foundations of bioethics. Boston (MA): Kluwer Academic Publishers; 1995. p. 131–47.

28. Sherwin S. No longer patient: feminist ethics and health care. Philadelphia (PA): Temple University Press; 1992.

29. Harlow NC, Killip T. Beyond do-not-resuscitate orders: a house staff mentoring and credentialing project on advance directives. Arch Intern Med 1997;157:135.

30. Tulsky JA, Fischer GS, Rose MR, Arnold RM. Opening the black box: how do physicians communicate about advance directives? Ann Intern Med 1998;129:441–9.

31. Miles SH, August A. Courts, gender and "the right to die." Law Med Health Care 1990;18:85–95.

Suggested Reading

American Medical Association. AMA Statement. Elements of quality care for patients in the last phase of life. Chicago (IL): AMA; 2003. Available at http://www.ama-assn.org/ama/pub/category/7567.html. Retrieved August 1, 2003.

American Medical Association. Code of medical ethics: current opinions with annotations. Chicago (IL): AMA; 2002.

American Medical Association. Reports on end-of-life care. Chicago (IL): AMA; 1998.

American Medical Association, The Robert Wood Johnson Foundation. EPEC: education for physicians on end-of-life care: participant's handbook. Chicago (IL): AMA; Princeton (NJ): RWJF; 1999.

Cassel CK, Foley KM. Principles for care of patients at the end of life: an emerging consensus among the specialties of medicine. New York (NY): Milbank Memorial Fund; 1999.

Dying well in the hospital: the lessons of SUPPORT. Hastings Cent Rep 1995;25(6):S1–36.

Joint Commission on Accreditation of Healthcare Organizations. Comprehensive accreditation manual for hospitals: the official handbook. Oakbrook Terrace (IL): JCAHO; 2000.

Quill TE. Caring for patients at the end of life: facing an uncertain future together. New York (NY): Oxford University Press; 2001.

Roberts JA, Brown D, Elkins T, Larson DB. Factors influencing views of patients with gynecologic cancer about end-of-life decisions. Am J Obstet Gynecol 1997;176:166–72.

Snyder L, Sulmasy DP, Ethics and Human Rights Committee, American College of Physicians-American Society of Internal Medicine. Physician-assisted suicide. Ann Intern Med 2001; 135:209–16.

Medical Futility

A proliferation in medical technology has dramatically increased the number of diagnostic and therapeutic options available in patient care. Health care costs also have increased as a byproduct of this technologic expansion. Simultaneously, medical ethics has undergone a rapid metamorphosis from a beneficence-focused ethic to one in which autonomy dominates: that is, from an ethic in which the physician always attempted to act for and in the best interest of the patient to one in which alternatives are presented to the patient and the patient makes the ultimate decision. Thus, not only the physician but also the patient may face the daunting task of selecting from among myriad highly technologic and expensive health care choices.

These, among other factors, have created situations in which patients or families have sometimes demanded care that physicians may deem "futile," or incapable of producing a desired result. The construct of medical futility has been used to justify a physician's unilateral refusal to provide treatment requested or demanded by a patient or the family of a patient. Such decisions may be based on the physician's perception of the inability of treatment to achieve a physiologic goal, to attain other goals of the patient or family, or to achieve a reasonable quality of life.

Although there is general agreement with the notion that physicians are not obligated to provide futile care (1), there is vigorous debate and little agreement on the definition of futile care, the appropriate determinants of each component of the definition, or who should be the agents whose values determine the definition of futility. Proposed definitions of medical futility require 1 or more of the following elements:

- The patient has a lethal diagnosis or prognosis of imminent death.
- Evidence exists that the suggested therapy cannot achieve its physiologic goal.
- Evidence exists that the suggested therapy will not or cannot achieve the patient's or family's stated goals.
- Evidence exists that the suggested therapy will not or cannot extend the patient's life span.
- Evidence exists that the suggested therapy will not or cannot enhance the patient's quality of life.

The following questions need to be addressed concerning each of the previously identified elements:

- What is imminent death? Is it death that is expected momentarily, or would it include death expected at any time up to 6 months or longer?
- What defines an inability to achieve the physiologic goal? Would it be that the goal could never be achieved or that the goal could be achieved in less than 1% of the cases, in 5% of the cases, or within some other established limit?
- What defines inability to achieve the patient's or family's goals?
- What is an enhanced life span—1 day, 1 week, 1 month?
- How is quality of life measured? Who determines what is a satisfactory quality of life?

As stakeholders in these determinations, agents (including patients, families, caregivers, and society as a whole) have an obligation to formulate these criteria. A patient may consider that even 1 more day of life is worth a therapeutic attempt or that living in a coma is more desirable than death.

Previously published as Committee Opinion 261, November 2001

A patient may consider that a 0.5% chance of stabilization after resuscitation warrants the effort. Physicians or society, however, may be less willing to provide the requested care as they balance the use of resources and their individual or collective view of potential benefit. Patients may not include the use of resources in their equation at all but simply balance negative side effects and risks versus potential beneficial outcome. Additionally, society may be more ready to accede to patient wishes when the use of resources is minimal than when it is significant, regardless of the likelihood of achieving physiologic goals, increasing life span, or achieving patient goals. Reasonableness and equity in the distribution of resources may play a role in determining whether societal and institutional values should prevail in contested decisions. When resource distribution is an issue, however, the values of the patient and the preservation of life ordinarily take priority and are ethical default positions.

Litigation also has generally supported the patient or family in cases in which patient and caregiver disagree regarding withholding care (2–6). Commentators have observed that court decisions in favor of patient or family wishes appear to be based on 1 of the following factors:

- Medicine's inability to define and quantify aspects of medical futility
- The lack of a prospective and clearly stated process for determining medical futility
- The courts' current bias toward autonomy
- A desire to be consistent in upholding the patient's rights whether the patient is refusing or requesting treatment

Need for a Medical Futility Policy

Inability to achieve a physiologic goal, or strict physiologic futility, is an appropriate basis for a physician to refuse to provide requested therapeutic intervention. However, it addresses only a limited number of clinical situations with medical futility conflicts.

Other interpretations of medical futility are too subjective to form the basis for unilateral physician decisions. Therefore, in the absence of strict physiologic futility, the construct of medical futility should be applied only according to a prospective organizational policy that provides a process rather than a rule for resolving conflict.

A policy would be valuable in those situations in which the probability of reaching a physiologic goal or the potential for enhancement of life's duration or quality is remote and there is disparity in the subjective interpretations by patient (family), physician, institution, and society regarding the cost (economic, physical, emotional)/benefit ratio. A medical futility policy should emphasize communication and negotiation rather than unilateral physician decision making and should be consistent with a published societal consensus on the use of resources, when available.

Designing a Medical Futility Policy

A medical futility policy should be built on the following foundations:

- It should be designed to enhance discussion among the parties.
- The responsible physician should be encouraged to involve all appropriate members of the treatment team (eg, house staff, nurses, social workers) to help reach an agreement between the patient (or surrogate) and the physician.
- It should be designed to enhance input from other individuals or groups with expertise in the relevant medical discipline or medical ethics (including clergy, attorneys, and ethics committees).
- It should allow a patient to select another caregiver whose view is more consistent with her own and facilitate transfer of care, without prejudice, by the original physician.
- If transfer of care is arranged, all life-sustaining treatment and interventions must be continued while the transfer is awaited.
- If no conciliation of views or patient transfer occurs, or if no other caregiver or facility is willing to provide the desired treatment, the caregivers are not required to provide care that they regard as medically futile.
- There must be some process of appeal as the situation comes closer to action by the physician or facility which is still contested by the patient or family.
- When caregivers refuse to provide a "futile intervention" or abrogate a certain aspect of treatment based on its futility, their obligation to provide care is undiminished. Providing comfort care and palliative care and maximizing quality of life at the end of life remain fundamental obligations of the physician responsible for a patient's care.

- The policy should require documentation that includes the following information:
  - Probable diagnoses
  - Probable prognosis
  - Physician-recommended alternatives
  - Patient-desired pathway
  - Process of decision making that was followed, including notes from relevant meetings

An example of a policy that provides a process for decision making in medical futility is outlined in the American Medical Association Council on Ethical and Judicial Affairs report, "Medical Futility in End-of-Life Care" (1) (Fig. 1).

Summary

It is difficult to define medical futility prospectively and objectively. Nonetheless, as technology continues to advance and use more resources, it is important that physicians and their institutions develop a process for dealing with conflict surrounding the construct of medical futility.

Prospective policies on medical futility are preferable to unilateral decision making by individual physicians. Such a medical futility policy should provide a systematic process for dealing with disagreements and for reaching a fair resolution, as outlined previously. When there is disagreement, patient and family values regarding treatment options and the default position of maintaining life ordinarily should take priority. However, situations

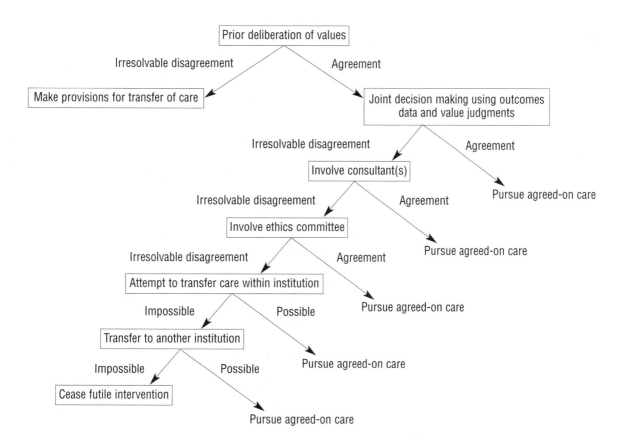

FIG. 1. Example of a process for considering futility cases. (Medical futility in end-of-life care: report of the Council on Ethical and Judicial Affairs. JAMA 1999;281:937–41. Copyright © 1999, American Medical Association. All rights reserved.)

may occur in which claims of reasonableness and equity in the distribution of resources are so powerful that the views of caregivers, the institution, and society will prevail.

References

1. Medical futility in end-of-life care: report of the Council on Ethical and Judicial Affairs. JAMA 1999;281:937–41.

2. Capron AM. In re Helga Wanglie. Hastings Cent Rep 1991;21(5):26–8.

3. Capron AM. Abandoning a waning life. Hastings Cent Rep 1995;25(4):24–6.

4. Angell M. The case of Helga Wanglie. A new kind of "right to die" case [letter]. N Engl J Med 1991;325:511–2.

5. Miles SH. Informed demand for "non-beneficial" medical treatment. N Engl J Med 1991;325:512–5.

6. Diekema DS. What is left of futility? The convergence of anencephaly and the Emergency Medical Treatment and Active Labor Act. Arch Pediatr Adolesc Med 1995;149:1156–9.

PART III

Professional Responsibilities

"To hold him who has taught me this art as equal to my parents and to live my life in partnership with him."—Hippocratic Oath (circa fourth century BCE)

As the 21st century unfolds with all its technologic advances, the concept of medicine as a profession persists. What duty do obstetrician–gynecologists owe to their present and future colleagues in the modern medical community? What obligations do they share in ensuring the continuation of the specialty and the pursuit of new medical knowledge?

This part of Ethics in Obstetrics and Gynecology *is focused on the relationship of obstetrician–gynecologists with their colleagues within the specialty and beyond. It offers ethical guidance on the formation of new specialists in obstetrics and gynecology. Consultation and referral relationships can advance the best interests of patients, and practical information is provided on establishing these relationships. Research poses special requirements, both ethical and regulatory, and these are addressed as well. Finally, other chapters address the fiduciary responsibilities of obstetrician–gynecologists to their patients and the ethical obligation not to abuse this trust.*

Obstetric–Gynecologic Education

Education of health care professionals is essential to maintain standards of competent and beneficial practice. Inherent in the education of health professionals is the problem of disparity in power and authority, including the power of teachers over students and the power of practitioners over patients* (1). It is therefore important to clarify both the professional responsibilities to those patients whose care provides educational opportunities and the responsibilities of teachers and students toward one another.

Ethical Responsibilities Toward Patients in Educational Settings

At the turn of the century, some medical educators were concerned about the needs of patients in "teaching hospitals," and they took steps to ensure that patients' rights would be protected. However, the prevailing opinion was more aptly characterized by a medical school faculty member: "Patients must clearly understand from the beginning that they are admitted for teaching purposes and that they are to be willing to submit to this when pronounced physically fit" (2). Unfortunately, this sentiment persists as an unstated presumption in some contemporary education programs. If the power inherent in the role of medical practitioner is misused in the educa-

Previously published as Committee Opinion 181, April 1996; content revised January 2004

*As commonly categorized by medical schools, residencies, and postgraduate fellowships, the learning and teaching roles of "student" and "teacher" represent a hierarchical approach to learning that does not reflect the reality of lifelong learning and teaching. The line between students and teachers in medicine is fluid and nonlinear. All clinicians learn from and teach each other at each point in the development of their profession. In this statement, the ethical obligations of teachers apply to all of those in the teaching role, wherever they may be in the educational continuum, and the obligations of students apply to all of those in the learning role.

tional setting, this misuse is likely to carry over into attitudes and relationships with future patients as well.

If health care professionals are to benefit society, they must be well educated and experienced. Acquisition of knowledge and skills in the educational process entails both benefits and risks. The benefits of health care to society provide the justification for exposure of patients to risks associated with education in clinical medicine. Although the benefits generally accrue to society at large, the burdens fall primarily on individual patients, especially the economically disadvantaged. These burdens are inherent in situations in which patients interact with students, for example, during medical histories, physical examinations, and diagnostic and surgical procedures.

Physicians must learn new skills and techniques in a manner consistent with the ethical obligations to benefit the patient, to do no harm, and to respect a patient's right to make informed decisions about health matters. These obligations must not be unjustifiably subordinated to the need and desire to learn new skills. In consideration of society's interest in the education of physicians, all patients should be considered "teaching patients." Race or socioeconomic status should not be the basis for selection of patients for teaching.

Although patients are given the opportunity to consent to or refuse treatment by students, the obligations of the profession, the institution, and patients should be made more uniform and explicit. Professional obligations include disclosure of the risks and benefits inherent in the teaching setting and provision of adequate supervision at all levels of training. The patient should be encouraged to participate in the teaching process to contribute her fair share to the development of a new generation of health care providers. A situation may arise in which a patient refuses, for whatever reason, to have a student involved in her health care. Such refusals should initiate discussion and counseling. Patient choice, however, must be handled with compassion and respect.

Some procedures, such as pelvic examinations, require specific consent. If a pelvic examination(s) that is planned for an anesthetized woman undergoing surgery offers her no personal benefit and is performed solely for teaching purposes, it should be performed only with her specific informed consent, obtained when she has full decision-making capacity.

Participation by anesthetized women in teaching exercises may be less common today than in the past. Alternatives to this training method exist that do not raise the challenges of securing informed consent. Today, many medical schools employ surrogates for patients to teach students how to perform pelvic examinations. These surrogates are variously referred to as gynecology teaching associates, professional patients, patient surrogates, standardized patients, or patient simulation. It is acknowledged, however, that in women preparing for surgery, the administration of anesthesia results in increased relaxation of the pelvic muscles, which may be beneficial in some educational contexts.

Finally, students must hold in confidence any information about patients learned in the context of a professional relationship. They should discuss specific patient care matters only in appropriate settings, such as teaching conferences or patient-management rounds. Conversations in public places, such as hospital corridors or elevators, involving comments about patients, their families, or the care they are receiving are inappropriate (3).

Ethical Responsibilities of Teachers to Students

The relationship between teacher and student in medical education inevitably involves the problem of imbalance of power and the risk of exploitation of a student for the benefit of the teacher (1). The teacher–student relationship exists at multiple levels among faculty members, medical students, attending physicians, fellows, and residents. Complex as it may be, there is a fundamental ethical responsibility at all levels for the teacher to impart wisdom, experience, and skill for the benefit of the student, without expectation of personal service by or reward from the student.

Because so much of medicine is learned in a preceptor–student relationship, great care must be taken that the teacher does not exploit the student. An example is the teacher who expects a student to spend time that is out of proportion to the educational value involved on a research project, but gives little or no credit for such a contribution. In this regard, the behavior of teachers toward students is a powerful example of ethics in action. Students are likely to model their behavior on that of their teachers (4).

The relationship of a teacher to a student involves not only trust and confidence but also power and dependency. It is the role of the teacher to foster independence in the student while nurturing the student in the learning process. This is a complex relationship, the boundaries of which can become obscured in the intense setting of clinical preceptorship (5). For example, the long hours spent by teachers and students in relatively arduous and isolated circumstances may foster amorous relationships. Regardless of the situation, the power imbalance makes a romantic or sexual relationship between a teacher and student ethically suspect. Amorous relationships between teachers and their current students are never appropriate.

Students should not be placed in situations where they must provide care or perform procedures for which they are not qualified and not adequately supervised. To do otherwise violates an ethical responsibility to the student as well as to the patient. A healthy relationship between teachers and students allows students to request assistance or supervision without fear of humiliation or retribution. Teaching should take place in an atmosphere that fosters mutual respect.

Conduct and Responsibilities of Students Toward Their Teachers

Students have the obligation to be honest, conscientious, and respectful in their relationships with their teachers. They should act in ways that preserve the dignity of patients and do not undermine relationships between patients and their physicians. It is the student's responsibility to ask for assistance and supervision when it is needed. Unfettered communication between student and teacher is essential in fostering an atmosphere that will allow, even encourage, students to request help. When such communication does not occur, both education and patient care suffer.

Inherent in the teacher–student relationship is the vulnerability of the student in dealing with perceived unethical behavior or incompetent conduct of a teacher. If a student observes such behavior or conduct, the matter should be brought to the attention of the appropriate institutional authority.

Institutional Responsibilities

Institutions have ethical obligations to students, patients, and teachers. Institutions have an obligation to provide a work environment that enhances professional competence. The health care system often has exploited students at all levels of education. Students may be viewed as a source of cheap labor, especially in busy hospitals on a teaching service. Students often provide long hours of service, and the resultant neglect of the student's physical and mental health must be balanced against the provision of an effective clinical experience. Lack of sleep, heavy workloads, and increasing amounts of responsibility without commensurate levels of authority are sources of great stress in medical education, especially during residency (6–8). The potentially negative impact of such an educational experience on the student's developing attitude toward patients and the profession should be considered. The obligation to provide a good work environment includes ensuring that students and residents work reasonable hours, establishing a balance between medical education and responsibility for patient care, providing adequate ancillary and administrative support services, and, in the case of residents, providing reasonable salaries and benefits (9).

A source of substantial stress for some students and residents is the conflict between family responsibilities and the demands of medical education (10). For many students, sleep deprivation resulting from long work hours results in fatigue, irritability, and anxiety. The inability to relate with consideration or affection to a partner or spouse or to participate in any effective way with child care or other domestic responsibilities may seriously impair family relationships. Also, with increasing numbers of women in education programs, special attention must be given to the parallel demands of pregnancy (including the postpartum period) and career goals. Providing ample time to sustain family relationships without adversely affecting the educational experience or imposing excessive burdens on colleagues is a daunting task, but one that must be confronted. Shared positions and more flexible time lines for completing educational requirements can be helpful in solving such problems.

Institutions should maintain a well-established reporting and review process for investigating allegations of unethical behavior or incompetent conduct. Access to such a process can facilitate fair and just relationships between students and teachers in these precarious situations.

As concerns about cost containment increase, education could become a low priority. The process of medical education may reduce the efficiency of patient care and increase costs. It is the responsibility of all physicians and institutions involved in the education of health care professionals to ensure that cost-reduction efforts do not diminish the opportunities for education in clinical medicine. Institutions have an ethical responsibility to develop policy statements and guidelines for the inclusion of students in patient care in ways that ensure sound medical education and high-quality medical care.

Conclusion

The effective education of students, residents, interns, fellows, and other professionals is essential if the health care professions are to benefit society. The power and authority inherent in relationships between students and patients as well as between teachers and students are important ethical concerns. Power and authority should be exercised responsibly to protect patients' dignity and welfare and to enhance the educational process.

Respect for autonomy requires that patients be informed about the extent to which students at any level are involved in their care and that patients' concerns be addressed. Students should provide only that level of care for which they are qualified and adequately supervised. Working conditions and work schedules should reflect a sensitivity for student welfare in its broadest terms. This attention to ethics will promote attitudes conducive to the compassionate and skilled treatment of patients. This emphasis also should serve as a model for the next generation of teachers.

References

1. Brody H. Medical ethics and power. In: The healer's power. New Haven (CT): Yale University Press; 1992. p. 12–25.
2. Ludmerer KM. Meaning of the teaching hospital. In: Learning to heal: the development of American medical education. New York (NY): Basic Books Inc; 1985. p. 231–3.
3. Ubel PA, Zell MM, Miller DJ, Fischer GS, Peters-Stefani D, Arnold RM. Elevator talk: observational study of inappropriate comments in a public space. Am J Med 1995; 99:190–4.

4. Bosk CL. Forgive and remember: managing medical failure. Chicago (IL): University of Chicago Press; 1979.

5. Plaut SM. Boundary issues in teacher-student relationships. J Sex Marital Ther 1993;19:210–9.

6. Butterfield PS. The stress of residency. A review of the literature. Arch Intern Med 1988;148:1428–35.

7. Stress and impairment during residency training: strategies for reduction, identification, and management. Resident Services Committee, Association of Program Directors in Internal Medicine. Ann Intern Med 1988; 109:154–61.

8. McCall TB. The impact of long working hours on resident physicians. N Engl J Med 1988;318:775–8.

9. Asch DA, Parker RM. The Libby Zion case. One step forward or two steps backward? N Engl J Med 1988; 318:771–5.

10. Green MJ. What (if anything) is wrong with residency overwork? Ann Intern Med 1995;123:512–7.

Seeking and Giving Consultation

Physicians have a long history of working together and with other health care professionals to provide efficient and comprehensive care for the patients they serve. Achieving these goals sometimes requires that physicians or other care providers seek consultation from or provide consultation to their colleagues (1). The basic principles of consultation for obstetrician–gynecologists are summarized in the "Code of Professional Ethics of the American College of Obstetricians and Gynecologists" as follows (see Appendix):

- "The obstetrician–gynecologist's relationships with other physicians, nurses, and health care professionals should reflect fairness, honesty, and integrity, sharing a mutual respect and concern for the patient."
- "The obstetrician–gynecologist should consult, refer, or cooperate with other physicians, health care professionals, and institutions to the extent necessary to serve the best interests of their patients."

Although consultation usually is requested in an efficient manner that expedites patient care, situations occur in which the relationship between practitioners or between institutions and practitioners results in an inefficient, less-than-collegial consultative process that may not be in the best interest of the patient. For example, a patient and a consultant may be put at serious disadvantage when consultation is requested late in the process of care or is not accompanied by sufficient background information or the reason for consultation is not clearly stated. Conversely, those seeking consultation may be denied assistance on arbitrary grounds. The present statement outlines the purpose of consultation and

referral, states the underlying ethical foundations that govern consultation and referral, and elaborates specifically the responsibilities of those who seek and those who provide consultation. This chapter is directed to physicians but it should be recognized that nonphysician practitioners also may be involved in consultation.

The Purpose of Consultation and Referral

Typically, a patient first seeks care from her primary caregiver (2), who should be aware that the patient's needs may go beyond his or her education, training, or experience (see Appendix) (3). Various levels of consultation may be needed to make correct diagnoses, provide technical expertise, and recommend a course of action (see box). Occasionally, consultation or referral may be indicated when a patient's request for care is in conflict with her primary caregiver's recommendations or preferences. Finally, a patient may seek consultation with another caregiver to obtain a second opinion or explore other options for care (4). In all of these types of consultation, the overriding principle is that consultation is primarily for the benefit of the patient (2).

Ethical Foundations

Ethical principles require that the consultative process be guided by the following concepts (see Appendix) (5):

- The welfare of the patient should be central to the consultant–patient relationship (beneficence).
- The patient should be fully informed about the need for consultation and participate in the selection of the consultant (autonomy).

Previously published as Committee Opinion 233, April 2000

Definitions: Levels of Consultation

Consultation is the act of seeking assistance from another physician(s) or health care professional(s) for diagnostic studies, therapeutic interventions, or other services that may benefit the patient. There are several levels of consultation (American College of Physicians Ad Hoc Committee on Medical Ethics, Kitchens LW. Ethics manual. 4th ed. Philadelphia [PA]: ACP; 1998. p. 35.):

- Informal consultation
- Single-visit consultation
- Continuing collaborative care
- Transfer of primary clinical responsibility

Informal consultation, in which the consultant does not talk with or examine the patient, usually involves a simple question from the referring practitioner that is answered by the consultant. The consultant does not make an entry in the patient's medical record or charge a fee, and the referring practitioner should not attribute an opinion to the consultant. Examples of informal consultations are questions regarding the significance of an irregular blood antibody or the follow-up interval for an abnormal Pap test. Such a consultation does not establish a patient–consultant relationship.

A single-visit consultation involves examination of the patient or the patient's medical record and performance of diagnostic tests or therapeutic procedures. The findings, procedures, and recommendations of the consultant are recorded in the patient's medical record or provided to the practitioner with primary clinical responsibility for the patient in a written report or letter, and a fee may be charged. The subsequent care of the patient continues to be provided by the referring practitioner. Examples of such consultations are confirming the findings of a pelvic examination, performing a specific urodynamic procedure on a patient with urinary stress incontinence, and interpreting an electronic fetal monitoring tracing or imaging studies. In the latter 2 cases, the tracing or other output can be transmitted electronically, allowing for the performance of a single-visit consultation without personal contact between the patient and consultant.

Continuing collaborative care describes a relationship in which the consultant provides ongoing care in conjunction with the referring practitioner. Thus, the consultant assumes at least partial responsibility for the patient's care. An example is a high-risk obstetric patient with a medical complication of pregnancy who is periodically assessed by the consultant, while the referring practitioner is responsible for the day-to-day management of the patient.

Transfer of primary clinical responsibility to the consultant may be appropriate for the management of problems outside the scope of the referring practitioner's education, training, and experience or in cases in which the patient must be transferred to another facility. Examples are the transfer of care of a patient in preterm labor from a birth center to a consultant in a perinatal center or referral of a patient with ovarian cancer to a gynecologic oncologist. In many of these situations, patients will eventually return to the care of the referring practitioner when the problem for which the consultation was sought is resolved.

- The patient should have access to adequate consultation regardless of her medical condition, social status, or financial situation (justice).
- Practitioners must disclose to patients any pertinent actual or potential conflict of interest that is involved in a consultation relationship, including financial incentives or penalties or restrictive guidelines (truth-telling).

In addition, both practitioners with primary clinical responsibility and consultants must respect the rights of the patient and also the rights of their respective professional colleagues.

Responsibilities Associated With Consultation

Seeking Consultation and Requesting Referral

Consultations usually are sought when practitioners with primary clinical responsibility recognize conditions or situations that are beyond their level of expertise or available resources. Historically, these practitioners acted as independent agents who decided when consultation was appropriate, determined the level of consultation, and were free to choose particular consultants. More recently, as a result of recognition of the importance of patient autonomy, practitioners now inform patients of the need for consultation and discuss options with them. The quality of the consultation often is improved by this collaborative relationship between practitioners and patients.

Today, this practitioner–patient partnership operates under new conditions that may affect the process of consultation. Under certain types of managed care arrangements, health care guidelines and protocols may limit the freedom of the practitioner to provide complete care or to request consultation (6). These guidelines may include instructions about specific situations or medical conditions in which consultation, second opinion, or referral is mandated (7). Examples include abnormal labor that may require operative delivery or chronic uterine bleeding that may require hysterectomy. Other guidelines may require that practitioners seek consultation when patients develop signs and symptoms of severe preeclampsia or if ovarian cancer is discovered. Such arrangements and guidelines may be designed to ensure a high level of care for patients by requiring that consultants be involved appropriately in certain clinical problems.

Conversely, practitioners may find themselves in situations that create disincentives to medically appropriate consultation or that mandate use of a consultant panel that is not adequate to support appropriate patient care. The policies that lead to such situations involve potential conflicts of interest (8) and may have a negative effect on the patient's medical needs, thus limiting her autonomy and her right to informed choice. Under all conditions of practice—solo or group, fee for service or managed care contract—consultation and referral should be carried out in the patient's best interest and obtained with the patient's consent after full disclosure of limitations and potential conflicts of interest.

It is in everyone's best interest—practitioners with primary clinical responsibility, consultants, patients, and health care plans—that the criteria for consultation be mutually agreed on in advance and stated clearly in writing. Financial incentives or penalties for consultation and referral that exist either overtly or covertly under many managed care contracts are sources of serious conflicts of interest. Practitioners must be free to inform patients of the best medical practice or options of care, even when the mandate of directed referrals under contracted care does not include these alternatives. Ethical responsibility for patients' best interests demands that practitioners disclose any proscriptions to serving as patients' advocates. Practitioners have a responsibility to provide patients with their best medical judgment and serve as advocates for patients if recommended care is denied. It then becomes the patients' responsibility to decide whether to abide by insurance plan restrictions, challenge them, or seek care outside the scope of coverage.

Giving Consultation and Accepting Referral

Physicians generally provide consultations or accept referred patients in the interest of providing excellent care for patients and promoting good relationships among colleagues. Open communication and established professional relationships facilitate effective consultation and referral. However, at times a consultant may be called on unexpectedly, inconveniently, and sometimes inappropriately to be involved in or to assume the care of a patient. In these situations, a physician is only ethically obligated to provide consultation or assume the care of the patient if there is a contractual agreement or a preexisting patient–physician relationship or if there is a severe medical emergency in which there is no reasonably available alternative caregiver (9). Hospital or departmental guidelines for consultation and referral may prevent such confrontations.

Practical Recommendations

Providing optimal care demands a good working relationship with a number of other physicians and health care professionals. Consultation may be needed by the practitioner with primary clinical responsibility regardless of specialty designation or level of training. Ideally, the referring practitioner–consultant relationship has been established before the need for consultation or referral arises, and the referring practitioner–consultant relationship should be ongoing.

One way to maximize prompt, effective consultation and collegial relationships is to have a formal consultation protocol. This may be especially advantageous for family physicians who provide obstetric or gynecologic care and for collaborative practice between obstetrician–gynecologists and nurse practitioners, certified nurse–midwives, and other health care professionals. Such protocols create pathways that anticipate difficult or complex situations.

Responsibilities of the Referring Practitioner

The responsibilities of the referring practitioner can be outlined as follows:

1. The referring practitioner should request consultation in a timely manner, whenever possible before an emergency arises. A good working relationship between the referring practitioner and consultant requires shared concern for the patient's needs and a commitment to timely and clear-cut communication.

2. The referring practitioner is responsible for preparing the patient with an explanation of the reasons for consultation, the steps involved, and the names of qualified consultants.

3. The referring practitioner should provide a summary of the history, physical examination, laboratory findings, and any other information that may facilitate the consultant's evaluation and recommendations (10).

4. Whenever possible, the referring practitioner should document in the medical record the indications for the consultation and specific issues to be addressed by the consultant.

5. The level of consultation (see "Definitions: Levels of Consultation" box) should be established by a dialogue between the referring practitioner and the consultant that results in mutual agreement.

Responsibilities of the Consultant

The responsibilities of the consultant can be outlined as follows:

1. Consultants should recognize their individual boundaries of expertise and provide only those medically accepted services and technical procedures for which they are qualified by education, training, and experience.

2. When asked to provide consultation, the consultant should do so in a timely manner and without regard to the specialty designation or qualifications of the referring practitioner. If the consultant believes that the referring practitioner is not qualified to provide an appropriate level of continuing care, the consultant should recommend to the referring practitioner and, if necessary, to the patient that the referring practitioner transfer care of the patient.

3. If a physician is asked to provide an "informal consultation" and believes an examination of the patient or her medical record is necessary to answer the question appropriately, the consultant may request the right to provide a formal consultation.

4. The consultant should effectively communicate findings, procedures performed, and recommendations to the referring practitioner at the earliest opportunity (4).

5. For all but informal consultations, a summary of the consultation should be included in the medical record or sent to the referring practitioner by letter or written report.

6. The extent to which the consultant will be involved in the ongoing care of the patient should be clearly established by mutual agreement of the consultant, the referring practitioner, and the patient. At times it may be appropriate for the consultant to assume primary clinical responsibility for the patient. Even if this is only a temporary circumstance, the consultant should obtain the referring practitioner's cooperation and assent whenever possible.

7. When the consultant does not have primary clinical responsibility for the patient, he or she should try to obtain concurrence for major procedures or additional consultants from the referring practitioner.

8. In all that is done, the consultant must respect the relationship between the patient and the referring practitioner, being careful not to diminish inappropriately the patient's confidence in her other caregivers (2).

9. The consultant should be cognizant of the referring practitioner's abilities. Reliance on these abilities may increase convenience to the patient, limit transportation needs, and ultimately result in more cost-effective care.

10. In the rare situation in which there is clear evidence that the patient's health is likely to be harmed by a continuing level of substandard care, the consultant has an obligation to discuss with the referring practitioner the problems that have been identified, recommend appropriate medical measures, and, when necessary, inform the patient.

A complex clinical situation may call for multiple consultations. Unless authority has been transferred elsewhere, the responsibility for the patient's care should rest with the referring practitioner (2). This practitioner should remain in charge of communication with the patient and coordinate the overall care on the basis of information derived from the consultants. This will ensure a coordinated effort that remains in the patient's best interest.

References

1. Referral of patients. In: American Medical Association Council on Ethical and Judicial Affairs. Code of medical ethics: current opinions with annotations. Chicago (IL): AMA; 2002. p. 106–7.
2. American College of Physicians Ad Hoc Committee on Medical Ethics, Kitchens LW. Ethics manual. 4th ed. Philadelphia (PA): ACP; 1998. p. 35.
3. American College of Obstetricians and Gynecologists. Physicians working with physicians. In: The assistant: information for improved risk management. Washington, DC: ACOG; 2001. p. 19–20.
4. Consultation. In: American Medical Association Council on Ethical and Judicial Affairs. Code of medical ethics: current opinions with annotations. Chicago (IL): AMA; 2002. p. 181.
5. Beauchamp TL, Childress JF. Principles of biomedical ethics. 5th ed. New York (NY): Oxford University Press; 2001.
6. Wallach EE, Fox HE, Gordon T, Faden R. Symposium: managed care and ethics. Contemp Ob Gyn 1998;43: 162–76.

7. Chervenak FA, McCullough LB, Chez RA. Responding to the ethical challenges posed by the business tools of managed care in the practice of obstetrics and gynecology. Am J Obstet Gynecol 1996;175:523–7.

8. Cain JM, Jonsen AR. Specialists and generalists in obstetrics and gynecology: conflicts of interest in referral and an ethical alternative. Women's Health Issues 1992;2: 137–45.

9. Free choice. In: American Medical Association Council on Ethical and Judicial Affairs. Code of medical ethics: current opinions with annotations. Chicago (IL): AMA; 2002. p. 255–7.

10. American College of Obstetricians and Gynecologists. Role of the obstetrician–gynecologist in the diagnosis and treatment of breast disease. ACOG Committee Opinion 186. Washington, DC: ACOG; 1997.

Institutional Responsibility To Provide Legal Representation

The "Code of Professional Ethics of the American College of Obstetricians and Gynecologists" states, "The obstetrician–gynecologist should strive to address through the appropriate procedures the status of those physicians who demonstrate questionable competence, impairment, or unethical or illegal behavior. In addition, the obstetrician–gynecologist should cooperate with appropriate authorities to prevent the continuation of such behavior."

Academic institutions, professional corporations, hospitals, and other health care organizations should have policies and procedures by which alleged violations of professional behavior can be reported and investigated. Also, it is necessary for these institutions to adopt policies on legal representation and indemnification for their employees or others acting in an official capacity who, in discharging their obligations relative to unethical or illegal behavior of individuals, are exposed to potential costly legal actions.

The American College of Obstetricians and Gynecologists agrees with the position of the American Association of University Professors in its 1995 statement, "Institutional Responsibility for Faculty Liability," that institutions should ensure effective legal and other necessary representation and full indemnification for any faculty member named or included in lawsuits or other legal proceedings arising from an act or omission in the discharge of institutional or professional duties (1).

Reference

1. Institutional responsibility for legal demands on faculty. American Association of University Professors. Academe 1999;85(1):52.

Previously published as Committee Opinion 204, July 1998

Commercial Enterprises in Medical Practice

Increasing financial pressures and the pervasiveness of entrepreneurial values in our society have led to an increase in the scope of activities for which physicians have sought reimbursement. As a result, increasing numbers of physicians sell and promote both medical and nonmedical products as part of their practices.

Physicians always have rendered advice and treatment for a fee, and this practice is appropriate; however, the sale and promotion of products for financial benefit is qualitatively different from these traditional activities. It is unethical under most circumstances for physicians to sell or promote medical or nonmedical products or services for their financial benefit. This chapter will examine the following issues:

- The scope of the inappropriate activities
- The reasons for their unacceptability
- The limited circumstances under which they may be acceptable

Recommendations

Sale or promotion of products by physicians to their patients is unethical, with some exceptions, in either clinical sites or other places. Sale or promotion of products by physicians to their patients is unethical whether conducted in person, by telephone, or by written solicitation. The following activities are considered unethical, subject to the exceptions outlined later in the chapter:

- Sale of prescription drugs to be used at home (For example, some commercial drug repackagers prepare these medicines in standard doses and provide them to physicians, who then resell them to patients [1].)

Previously published as Committee Opinion 254, April 2001

- Sale or promotion of nonprescription medicine
- Sale or promotion of presumptively therapeutic agents that generally are not accepted as part of standard medical practice
- Sale or promotion of non-health-related items, such as household supplies (2)
- Recruitment of patients or of other health care professionals into multilevel marketing arrangements (These are enterprises in which individuals recruit other individuals to sell products and receive a commission on sales by their recruits. These recruits, in turn, can recruit a third generation of marketers, whose commissions are shared with participants of earlier generations.)
- Sale or promotion of any product in whose sale the physician has a significant financial interest, even if the sale would otherwise be appropriate (Such financial interest includes, among other things, sale for a direct profit, or sale of a product in whose manufacturer or wholesaler the physician holds a substantial equity interest [3].)

Exceptions

Circumstances in which it is ethical and appropriate to sell products to patients are as follows:

- Sales of devices or drugs that require professional administration in the office setting (Under these circumstances, the charge for the product should not exceed the costs, which may include both the direct cost of the product and the overhead incurred in obtaining, storing, and administering it.)
- Sales of therapeutic agents, when no other facilities can provide them at reasonable convenience and at reasonable cost (This circumstance might occur in a thinly populated area or in a locality in which certain forms of reproductive control are

unpopular. If physicians sell such products, the price charged should not exceed the cost of the product, including both direct and overhead costs.)

- Sales that clearly are external to the patient–physician relationship, when such sales ordinarily would be considered appropriate in the context of an external relationship (An example of such a transaction is a brokered house sale at a fair market price.)
- Sales of low-cost products for the benefit of community organizations (An example of such a product is Girl Scout cookies. These products must be sold without pressure, and the physician must not derive a profit from such sales.)

Rationale

There have been arguments given to support the sale in physicians' offices of drugs and other products related to the treatment of patients (1). One is convenience—a busy patient need not go to a pharmacy. Another, although not borne out by empirical studies, is that increasing the number of dispensers of drugs reduces the cost of drugs (1). Finally, it is possible that adherence to treatment is improved if the patient purchases the drug from the physician.

Under most circumstances, however, the sale of products by physicians violates several generally accepted principles of medical ethics. First, and most important, the practice of physician sales to patients creates a potential conflict of interest with the physician's fiduciary responsibility to provide "a right and good healing action taken in the interests of a particular patient" (4). This principle of fidelity is defined as the obligation of physicians to put the interests of patients above their own.

Physicians must not engage in actions that violate or call into question their fiduciary relationship with patients. The term *conflict of interest* refers to circumstances in which this commitment to the fiduciary relationship is compromised. Conflict of interest contains 2 elements: "1) an individual with an obligation, fiduciary or otherwise, and 2) the presence of conflicting interests that may undermine fulfillment of the obligation" (5).

The American Medical Association (AMA) and other professional societies have long opposed practices that result in conflicts of interest, with AMA's Council on Ethical and Judicial Affairs (CEJA) stating that "as professionals, physicians are expected to devote their energy, attention and loyalty fully to the service of their patients" (6). Many statements issued by CEJA and other AMA bodies have condemned various practices resulting in conflict of interest. These related improper commercial practices include fee splitting (payment by or to a physician solely for the referral of a patient), physician self-referral, physician ownership of pharmacies, and selling medical products (7). They have condemned physician ownership of stock in laboratories that pay physicians in proportion to the amount of work they refer, as well as disapproving of rebates from optical or medical instrumentation companies (5, 8).

Referral by physicians to health care facilities, such as laboratories, in which they do not engage in professional activities but in which they have a financial interest is called *self-referral*. This practice is analogous to product sales in that physicians are deriving a profit from goods (eg, laboratory tests or drugs) that they did not produce. Both of these practices create a clear conflict of interest because referring physicians accept money from vendors to direct patients to use their products or services instead of alternative products or services (including the option of no treatment at all). The conflict, therefore, is between the financial advantage that accrues from physicians' sales or referrals and physicians' obligation to arrange the best possible ancillary and consultative services for their patients. For example, CEJA states that self-referral to outside facilities is ethical only "if there is a demonstrated need in the community for the facility and alternative financing is not available" (6). In these circumstances, the practice is considered ethical only if referring physicians meet certain requirements designed to ensure that they receive no more financial consideration than would an ordinary investor and that certain safeguards are taken to avoid exploitation of patients.

Several other cardinal principles are violated by the practice of sales by physicians. The principle of truthfulness is violated if a conflict of interest related to the sale exists and is not communicated to the patient.

The principle of nonmaleficence is violated when there is potential injury to patients, which could occur in several ways. Physicians may be tempted to sell to patients items that they do not need. Even if its use is appropriate, the product in question may not be the most suitable for given patients. For example, joint ventures in radiation oncology (ie, those in which referring physicians had a financial interest) were found to provide more frequent and more intense use of radiation therapy than did freestanding facilities, without increased benefit (9).

Another principle that may be violated by this practice is that of autonomy. A patient who might otherwise elect to compare various alternatives to the product sold by the physician on whom she depends for advice and treatment could feel constrained to accept the physician's product. She may feel coercion to comply with treatments with which she does not agree. If the product is not health related, patients might feel constrained to purchase goods they do not want (8).

Finally, this practice violates the principles of professionalism and professional solidarity by weakening public trust in the profession. As CEJA has stated, "The medical profession's ability to preserve autonomy and the nature of the physician–patient relationship during periods of transformation have succeeded in large part due to the profession's lack of tolerance for 'commercialism' in medicine" (6).

Conclusion

The sale or promotion of products by physicians to their patients rarely is ethical. Exceptions have been described in this chapter. Practitioners of obstetrics and gynecology should not engage in commercial arrangements that result in real, apparent, or potential conflicts of interest.

References

1. James DN. Selling drugs in the physician's office. Bus Prof Ethics J 1992;11:73–88.
2. Rice B. What's a doctor doing selling Amway? Med Econ 1997;74:79–82, 85–6, 88.
3. Responsibility of applicants for promoting objectivity in research for which PHS funding is sought. 42 C.F.R. §50 Subpart F (2002).
4. Pellegrino ED, Thomasma DC. A philosophical reconstruction of medical morality. In: A philosophical basis of medical practice: toward a philosophy and ethic of the healing professions. New York (NY): Oxford University Press; 1981. p. 192–220.
5. Rodwin MA. The organized American medical profession's response to financial conflicts of interest: 1890–1992. Milbank Q 1992;70:703–41.
6. Conflicts of interest. Physician ownership of medical facilities. Council on Ethical and Judicial Affairs, American Medical Association. JAMA 1992;267:2366–9.
7. Sale of health-related products from physicians' offices. In: American Medical Association Council on Ethical and Judicial Affairs. Code of medical ethics: current opinions with annotations. Chicago (IL): AMA; 2002. p. 204–5.
8. Sale of non-health-related goods from physicians' offices. Council on Ethical and Judicial Affairs, American Medical Association. JAMA 1998;280:563.
9. Mitchell JM, Sunshine JH. Consequences of physicians' ownership of health care facilities—joint ventures in radiation therapy. N Engl J Med 1992;327:1497–501.

Research Involving Women

Attitudes concerning inclusion of women in research trials have changed dramatically over the past 3 decades. In the 1970s and 1980s, women were systematically excluded from participating in research trials either because of the fear that unrecognized pregnancy might place an embryo at risk or because a uniform all-male sample would simplify analysis of data. In addition, pregnant women were excluded from most research trials because they were viewed as a vulnerable population requiring special protection, and there was concern that trial participation would result in harm to the fetus. Another fear was that participation of pregnant women in research trials would result in increased liability risk for researchers. In the past decade, there has been a dramatic policy shift toward wide-scale inclusion of women in research trials. This policy shift is a direct result of a conscious effort by government agencies to expand participation of women in research in order to obtain valid, evidence-based information about health and disease in this population (1).

This chapter is designed to provide reasonable guidelines for research involving women. In this chapter, the American College of Obstetricians and Gynecologists' Committee on Ethics affirms both the need for women to serve as research subjects and the obligation for researchers, institutional review boards (IRBs), and others reviewing clinical research to evaluate the potential effect of proposed research on women of childbearing potential, pregnant women, and the developing fetus.

Rationale for Including Women in Research

All women should be presumed to be eligible for participation in clinical studies. The potential for pregnancy should not automatically exclude a woman from participating in a clinical study, although contraception may be required for participation. Inclusion of women in clinical studies is necessary for valid inferences about health and disease in women. The generalization to women of results from trials conducted in men may yield erroneous conclusions that fail to account for the biologic differences between men and women.

The rationale for conducting research in women is to advance knowledge in the following areas:

- Medical conditions in women (eg, cardiovascular disease)
- Physiology of women
- Sex differences in responses to drugs (eg, antiretroviral agents)
- Sex differences in drug toxicities
- Sex differences in responses to disease (eg, mental disorders)
- Effects of hormonal contraceptives on response to other therapies (eg, seizure medication)
- Variations in response to therapy at different stages of the menstrual cycle and the life cycle

The rationale for conducting research in pregnant and postpartum women is to advance knowledge in the following areas:

- Medical conditions (eg, human immunodeficiency virus [HIV]) in women who become pregnant
- Medical conditions unique to pregnancy (eg, preeclampsia)
- Conditions that threaten the successful course of pregnancy (eg, preterm labor)
- Prenatal conditions that might threaten the health of the fetus (eg, diaphragmatic hernia)
- Physiologic changes that accompany pregnancy and lactation

Previously published as Committee Opinion 290, November 2003

- Medical conditions related to pregnancy that might affect the future health of women (eg, gestational diabetes)
- Safety of medication during pregnancy and breastfeeding

Human experimentation is a necessary and important part of biomedical research because certain information can be obtained in no other way. Guidelines for protection of research participants have been established and are applicable to women of childbearing potential as well as to pregnant women (2–4). Additional protections have been established for pregnant women (5, 6). Participants in research should expect full disclosure of the burdens and benefits of the research study and should understand the potential risks as well as benefits. Investigators must use research design methods that employ means to maximize safety and minimize risk. A fully informed consent process and review of study protocols by IRBs act as safeguards to ensure that efforts to increase access to and participation of women in clinical trials will not result in procedural shortcuts that violate basic ethical standards.

Involvement in research protocols should not diminish a woman's expectation that she will receive appropriate medical care during the study and in the future. Health care professionals have a responsibility to provide the most appropriate clinical management, whether or not a woman is a participant in research. Research objectives should not affect clinical management. If a conflict arises between medically appropriate patient care and research objectives, patient care should prevail. For example, it is inappropriate to attempt to delay a medically indicated induction of labor solely to meet gestational age criteria for participation in a research project. The welfare of the patient and, in the case of pregnancy, the patient and her fetus is always the primary concern.

The Ethical Context

Ethical Requirements for Research

To be considered ethically justified, research on human subjects must satisfy several conditions. These include a reasonable prospect that the investigation will produce the knowledge that is being sought, a favorable balance of benefits over risks, a proven necessity to use human subjects, a system for independent monitoring of outcomes and protection of human subjects, and a fair allocation of the burdens and benefits of the research among potential subject groups (7). These principles should not be weakened by attempts to increase participation of women in research trials.

Although it is important to try to distinguish ethical problems involving patient care from ethical issues related to research, a definitive line cannot always be drawn between the 2 areas. The dual role that physicians often assume as research scientists and clinical practitioners may result in conflict of interest, because each role has different goals and priorities. For example, the goal of the investigator is to generate knowledge that has the potential to benefit patients in the future, whereas clinicians are expected to act in the best interests of their current patients. Researchers need to recognize these potential problems, strive to resolve them before beginning specific research projects, and inform patients about potential conflicts as they seek consent for research participation.

The potential for role conflict becomes readily apparent when innovative therapies are introduced. In the context of maternal–fetal surgery, for example, innovative surgical procedures have been conducted, but the long-term impact on both the woman and the fetus is unclear. Some clinicians believe, based on their experience, that in utero repair of myelomeningocele results in a better long-term prognosis for the infant than postnatal repair (8, 9). However, current data do not support this contention (10). In this context, it is important to conduct rigorous scientific evaluation of maternal–fetal surgery before this innovative therapy is offered as routine care.

Ethical Principles Supporting the Inclusion of Women

The recent movement to enroll more women in clinical research can be justified by ethical principles: beneficence, nonmaleficence, autonomy, and justice. Because disease processes may have different characteristics in women and men and because women and men may respond differently to treatments and interventions, women need to be included as subjects in clinical research. For women to benefit from the results of research (beneficence), the research must be designed to provide a valid analysis as to whether women are affected differently from men (1). Such differential analysis is necessary not only to benefit women, but also to prevent harm; if data from studies with men are inappropriately extrapolated to women, women may actually suffer harm (nonmaleficence).

Arguments previously advanced to defend the exclusion of women from research often cited the possibility of harms to women of reproductive potential or to pregnant women and their fetuses, harms that did not apply to men. However, the risk of such harms can be minimized and, in itself, does not justify the exclusion of women from research that is needed to make valid inferences about the medical treatment of women.

Because of their physical and physiologic characteristics, women have frequently been regarded as a vulnerable population that needs to be protected. Today, however, both civil society and medical ethics recognize the right and the capacity of women to make decisions regarding their own lives and their medical care (autonomy). Similarly, women have the right and the capacity to weigh the risks and potential benefits of participation in research and to decide for themselves whether to consent to participate. This autonomy right is limited, however, by the right of investigators and IRBs to take precautions to limit the risk for pregnant women and their fetuses.

Systematic exclusion of women from research violates the ethical principle of justice, which first requires that persons be given what is due them. If the medical treatment of women is invalidly based on studies that excluded women, then women are not receiving fair treatment. Justice requires that women be included in clinical studies in sufficient numbers to determine whether their responses are different from those of men.

In the research setting, justice requires that the benefits of scientific advancement be shared fairly between men and women. Both women and men should be encouraged to participate in research. Researchers should specifically address those obstacles to participation that are experienced disproportionately by women—for example, problems obtaining and paying for adequate child care during time spent as a research subject.

Because of a history of systematic exclusion of women from research, in 1993 Congress directed that women were to be included in all federally funded research projects (11). Consequently, the National Institutes of Health (NIH) now require that women be included in all NIH-funded clinical research, unless a clear and compelling rationale establishes that such involvement would be inappropriate or unsafe (1). Particular focus on the health needs of women is justifiable at this time in view of a history of neglect of such studies.

Informed Consent

Appropriate and adequately informed consent by the potential subject or another authorized person and an independent review of the risks and benefits of research by appropriate institutions or agencies (or both) are fundamental to the formulation of any research protocol (12). The informed consent process should not be weakened to benefit the researcher. The consent document should be understandable and written in simple language. In situations in which English is not the primary language of the potential study subject, an interpreter should be used for the consent process to verify the participant's level of understanding of the issues related to risk and benefit. The statement of informed consent may need to be translated into the subject's native language. Researchers should be familiar with federal and state laws and regulations for informed consent in settings where pregnant minors and adolescents are potential subjects for recruitment (13).

The researcher has an obligation to disclose to and discuss with the woman all material risks affecting her; in the case of a pregnant woman, this includes all material risks to the woman and her fetus (14). Disclosure should include risks that are likely to affect the patient's decision to participate or not to participate in the research. Because the process of informed consent cannot anticipate all conceivable risks, women who develop unanticipated complications should be instructed to contact the researcher or a representative of the IRB immediately. Pregnant women who enroll in a research trial and experience a research-related injury should be informed about their therapeutic options, including those related to the pregnancy.

The potential participant should be encouraged to consult her physician independently before deciding to participate in a research study (15). At the woman's request, the researcher should provide information about the study to her physician. If relevant, this information may include the requirements of the study and its possible outcomes and complications.

Both the researcher and the primary caregiver should guard against inflating the patient's perception of the therapeutic benefit expected from participating in the study. Studies have shown that research subjects tend to believe, despite careful explanation of research protocols, that they will always benefit from participation or that the level of actual benefit will be greater than stated in the consent process (16). This risk of "therapeutic misconception" may be increased when the patient's own physician is involved in the consent process, especially when one physician serves as both researcher and clinician.

Consent of the pregnant woman alone is sufficient for most research. When research has the prospect of direct benefit to the fetus alone, paternal consent also may be required (see Table 1). Federal regulations that call for involvement of the father in the consent process for research intended to benefit the fetus are controversial and have generated vigorous debate. Proponents of paternal consent endorse this requirement because they believe that the requirement is consistent with recognition of and respect for the rights of the father in protecting the welfare of his unborn child. They believe that this represents a reasonable compromise between acknowledging paternal rights and reducing barriers to participation in research by pregnant women.

The Committee on Ethics, however, does not support recognition of distinct paternal rights before the birth of a child. Recognition of paternal rights during pregnancy may infringe on and weaken maternal autonomy—the right of a woman, when pregnant, to independent action in decisions that affect her body and her health. As in clinical situations, the pregnant woman's consent should be sufficient for research interventions that affect her or her fetus. To further complicate matters, the interpretation as to whether research is intended for the benefit of the pregnant woman, the fetus, or both

may be subjective. Two researchers conducting identical studies may reach totally different conclusions as to whether benefits of the research apply to the pregnant woman, the fetus, or both (eg, maternal–fetal surgery for spina bifida).

Informed consent means that women have the right to choose not to participate in a research protocol and the right to withdraw from a study at any time. The participation of a woman in a research study is based on the expectation that she will consider carefully her own interests. The participation of a pregnant woman in a research study is based on the expectation that she will consider carefully her own interests as well as those of her fetus. Typically, pregnant women are quite willing to take personal risks for the benefit of their fetuses; combined with society's expectation that they will do so, women may find themselves under pressure to participate in research that carries risk to them. Such pressure actually may interfere with the ability of the pregnant woman to give fully free consent. In these situations, special care should be taken to ensure that a woman's consent is truly voluntary.

Research Related to Diagnosis and Therapy

Research that consists of observation and recording without clinical intervention (descriptive research) is of ethical concern primarily to the extent that it requires informed consent and the preservation of confidentiality. In research trials, where clinical

Table 1. Federal Regulations on Informed Consent for Participants in Human Research

Federal regulations on protection of human research subjects are found in the *Code of Federal Regulations* in Title 45, Part 46. Selected sections of the regulations dealing with informed consent are reprinted here; the complete, current version may be found at http://ohrp.osophs.dhhs.gov/humansubjects/guidance/45cfr46.htm.

Issue	Citation	Regulation
Maternal consent	45 C.F.R. §46.204(d)	If the research holds out the prospect of direct benefit to the pregnant woman, the prospect of a direct benefit both to the pregnant woman and the fetus, or no prospect of benefit for the woman nor the fetus when risk to the fetus is not greater than minimal and the purpose of the research is the development of important biomedical knowledge that cannot be obtained by any other means, her consent is obtained in accord with the informed consent provisions of subpart A* of this part;
Paternal consent	45 C.F.R. §46.204(e)	If the research holds out the prospect of direct benefit solely to the fetus then the consent of the pregnant woman and the father is obtained in accord with the informed consent provisions of subpart A* of this part, except that the father's consent need not be obtained if he is unable to consent because of unavailability, incompetence, or temporary incapacity or the pregnancy resulted from rape or incest.

*Basic U.S. Department of Health and Human Services policy for protection of human research subjects. 45 C.F.R. §46 Subpart A (2002).

intervention is a component, the benefits and burdens of the trial must be clearly articulated to the participant by the researcher (14). In research studies conducted in pregnant women, both the potential benefit to the woman, the fetus, and society as a whole and the level of risk that may be incurred as a result of participation in the study should be considered. The involvement of the participant's obstetrician is ordinarily appropriate. All parties concerned need to strive for clear communication with regard to the following questions:

- Does the research involve intervention or diagnosis that might affect the woman's or the fetus's well-being, or is the goal of the study to produce scientific results that will be likely to be useful to future patients but offer no demonstrable benefit to current subjects?
- Can the prospective subject expect any explicit benefit as a result of participating in the study? If not, she must be apprised of this fact. Those studies that search for general information and are not associated with diagnostic or treatment modalities would be less likely to create the impression that the research will result in direct benefit to the participant. The researcher is still obligated to verify that the subject has understood this aspect of the study correctly.
- Is there more than "minimal risk" to the fetus generated by the research?

According to applicable federal regulations, "minimal risk means that the probability and magnitude of harm or discomfort anticipated in the research are not greater in and of themselves than those ordinarily encountered in daily life or during the performance of routine physical or psychological examinations or tests" (17). It has been questioned whether the "daily life" used for comparison should be that of the general population or that of the subject. Using the participant's daily life as the standard might make a higher level of risk acceptable; therefore, the general population standard is advised (12). Anything beyond minimal risk must be weighed carefully against the potential benefits to the woman and the fetus when the advisability of participation is considered.

It is appropriate for investigators and sponsors, with the approval of the IRB, to require a negative pregnancy test result as a criterion for participation in research when the research may pose more than minimal risk to the fetus. For an adolescent, the process of informed consent should include a discussion about pregnancy testing and the management of pregnancy test results, including whether the results will be shared with her parents or guardian.

Similarly, it is reasonable for investigators and research sponsors, with the IRB's approval, to require effective birth control measures for women of reproductive capacity as an inclusion criterion for participation in research that may entail more than minimal risk to the fetus. Consultation with an obstetrician–gynecologist or other knowledgeable professional is encouraged if questions arise about efficacy and risk of contraceptive measures. When a fetus has been exposed to risk in the conduct of research, the woman should be strongly encouraged to participate in follow-up evaluations to assess the impact on the fetus.

After informed discussion about the research trial, some women will decline to participate. Researchers should respect this decision and not allow patient refusal to affect subsequent clinical care. Reasonable compensation for a woman's time, effort, and expense as a participant in a research study is both acceptable and desired, but researchers should not offer inducements, financial or otherwise, to influence participation in research beyond reasonable compensation for the woman's time, effort, and expense.

Recommendations of the Committee on Ethics

The Committee on Ethics makes the following recommendations for research involving women. In addition, federal and state laws and regulations governing research in this population should be observed (2, 5, 13):

1. Women should be presumed to be eligible for participation in all clinical studies except for those addressing health concerns solely relevant to men.
2. Women should be included in research in sufficient numbers to ensure that inferences from a clinical trial apply validly to both sexes.
3. All research on women should be conducted in a manner consistent with the following ethical principles:
   —It should conform to general scientific standards for valid research.
   —Research may be conducted only with the informed consent of the woman.
   —Researchers should not offer inducements, financial or otherwise, to influence participa-

tion in research beyond reasonable compensation for the woman's time, effort, and expense.

—Conscientious efforts should be made to avoid any conflicts between appropriate health care and research objectives. Health care needs of the individual woman should take precedence over research interests in all situations affecting clinical management.

4. Research involving pregnant women should conform to the following recommendations:

—Research may be conducted only with the informed consent of the woman. Pregnant women considering a research study should determine the extent to which the father is to be involved in the process of informed consent and the decision.

—Informed consent of the father must be obtained when federal regulations require it for research that has the prospect of direct benefit to the fetus alone.

—Research protocols should be evaluated for their potential impact on both the woman and the fetus, and that evaluation should be made as part of the process of informed consent.

In this chapter, an attempt has been made to take into account protection of human subjects, the eligibility of women to participate in research, and the benefits that society could derive from participation of women in research. These potential benefits include reduction in morbidity and mortality from sex-specific disease processes, as well as reduction in fetal, infant, and maternal mortality and morbidity.

References

1. National Institutes of Health. NIH policy and guidelines on the inclusion of women and minorities as subjects in clinical research, amended October 2001. Bethesda (MD): NIH; 2001. Available at http://grants.nih.gov/grants/funding/women_min/guidelines_amended_10_2001.htm. Retrieved May 27, 2003.
2. Protection of human subjects. 45 C.F.R. §46 (2002).
3. United States. National Commission for the Protection of Human Subjects of Biomedical and Behavioral Research. The Belmont Report: ethical principles and guidelines for the protection of human subjects of research. Washington, DC: U.S. Government Printing Office; 1978.
4. World Medical Association. Declaration of Helsinki: ethical principles for medical research involving human subjects. 52nd WMA General Assembly, Edinburgh, Scotland, October 2000. Bethesda (MD): National Institutes of Health; 2000. Available at http://206.102.88.10/ohsrsite/guidelines/helsinki.html. Retrieved May 28, 2003.
5. Additional protections for pregnant women, human fetuses and neonates involved in research. 45 C.F.R. §46 Subpart B (2002).
6. Research on transplantation of fetal tissue. Informed consent of donor. 42 U.S.C. §289g-1(b) (2000).
7. Beauchamp TL. The intersection of research and practice. In: Goldworth A, Silverman W, Stevenson DK, Young EW, Rivers R, editors. Ethics and perinatology. New York (NY): Oxford University Press; 1995. p. 231–44.
8. Bruner JP, Tulipan N, Paschall RL, Boehm FH, Walsh WF, Silva SR, et al. Fetal surgery for myelomeningocele and the incidence of shunt-dependent hydrocephalus. JAMA 1999;282:1819–25.
9. Sutton LN, Adzick NS, Bilaniuk LT, Johnson MP, Crombleholme TM, Flake AW. Improvement in hindbrain herniation demonstrated by serial fetal magnetic resonance imaging following fetal surgery for myelomeningocele. JAMA 1999;282:1826–31.
10. Neural tube defects. ACOG Practice Bulletin No. 44. American College of Obstetricians and Gynecologists. Obstet Gynecol 2003;102:203–13.
11. NIH Revitalization Act of 1993, Pub. L. No. 103-43 (1993).
12. United States. National Bioethics Advisory Commission. Ethical and policy issues in research involving human participants. Report and recommendations of the National Bioethics Advisory Commission. Vol. 1. Bethesda (MD): NBAC; 2001.
13. Additional protections for children involved as subjects in research. 45 C.F.R. §46.401–409 Subpart D (2002).
14. General requirements for informed consent. 45 CFR §46.116 (2002).
15. Institute of Medicine (US). Women and health research: ethical and legal issues of including women in clinical studies. Vol. 1. Washington, DC: National Academy Press; 1994. p. 175–202.
16. Appelbaum PS, Roth LH, Lidz CW, Benson P, Winslade W. False hopes and best data: consent to research and the therapeutic misconception. Hastings Cent Rep 1987;17: 20–4.
17. Definitions. 45 C.F.R. §46.102 (2002).

Preembryo Research

Research on the **preembryo*** has been surrounded with ethical questions for many years. These questions remain important because of the potential benefits to be gained from the research and the ongoing urgency of the ethical concerns both for and against it. This chapter does not assume the resolution of all debate on these questions; it acknowledges the diversity of ethical opinions among the members of the American College of Obstetricians and Gynecologists (ACOG) as among others in society at large. Positions range from complete rejection of all human preembryo research to approval of generating preembryos solely for research. Even among those who accept preembryo research on ethical grounds, there is disagreement about the conditions under which it may be carried out ethically. The purpose of this chapter is to present relevant considerations from the findings of contemporary embryology and to propose ethical guidelines for research.

Historical Perspective: Restrictions and Policies

In 1974, the U.S. Congress established the National Commission for the Protection of Human Subjects of Biomedical and Behavioral Research. The commission recommended and the government adopted guidelines for National Institutes of Health funding of fetal research. In 1975, a federal regulation was adopted stating that "No application or proposal involving human in vitro fertilization may be funded by the Department [now Health and Human Services] or any component thereof until the application or proposal has been reviewed by the Ethical Advisory Board and the Board has rendered advice

Previously published as Committee Opinion 136, April 1994
*Terms defined in the glossary are shown in bold print.

as to its acceptability from an ethical standpoint" (1). Consequently, a national Ethics Advisory Board (EAB) was established to review in vitro fertilization (IVF) research protocols and certain protocols for fetal research. In May 1978, the EAB agreed to review the ethics, legality, safety, efficacy, and scientific merit of IVF research receiving National Institutes of Health support. In a May 4, 1979, report, the EAB agreed that "the human embryo is entitled to profound respect; but this respect does not necessarily encompass the full legal and moral rights attributed to persons" (2). The EAB statement supported research on the safety and efficacy of IVF and embryo transfer techniques to be used for the treatment of infertility. The EAB recommended allowing the use of **gametes** of informed and consenting **donors** to study the safety and efficacy of clinical IVF, provided that developing human cells not be sustained longer than 14 days in vitro. By 1994, these recommendations had yet to be approved by the Secretary of Health and Human Services. In 1980, the EAB ceased to exist because of the Administration's unwillingness to appoint new members. Thus, as of 1994, no federal support of IVF research had been permitted.

Despite the moratorium on federal funding for IVF research in the United States, private and university-based research has proceeded in the context of infertility treatment. The American Fertility Society (AFS) (currently the American Society for Reproductive Medicine) Committee on Ethics recognized the ethical dilemmas implicit in IVF research and recommended specific guidelines for conducting such research. The AFS noted that the preembryonic stage is considered to last until 14 days after **fertilization**. The AFS Committee on Ethics, in its 1986 and 1990 reports, recommended that human preembryos not be maintained for research beyond the 14th day after fertilization (3, 4). A 14-day limit also was recognized by the EAB in 1979, the Waller Commission Report (Victoria, Australia) in 1984 (5), and the Warnock Committee Report (Great Britain) in 1984 (6).

In the absence of a national consensus, the climate in the United States has been influenced by these generally prudent and conservative recommendations. In 1991, the National Advisory Board on Ethics in Reproduction was established within the private sector. Among its goals, according to the board's statement of purpose, are providing a forum for public discussion and reviewing "such issues as in vitro fertilization research, research with early human embryos, research on preimplantation genetic diagnosis, and fetal tissue transplantation research."

Efforts to move forward with human preembryo research, then, have almost always been accompanied by a recognition of the need to deliberate about ethical problems and guidelines. Deliberations in this regard often have included a weighing of the importance of the research in relation to its risks to individuals and society and in relation to varying perceptions of the moral status of the preembryo.

The Benefits and Risks of Human Preembryo Research

Potential Benefits

The goals and objectives of preembryo research are numerous, varied, and—at least in some cases—relatively uncontroversial. They include, for example, the following goals and objectives:

- Increasing knowledge about embryogenesis and embryopathy
- Developing a better understanding of the biology of human **implantation**
- Understanding better the causes of spontaneous abortion
- Developing more effective or simpler forms of contraception
- Improving methods of IVF treatment for both male and female infertility
- Developing preembryo biopsy techniques for a preimplantation diagnosis of genetic or chromosomal abnormalities by new technologies such as DNA amplification
- Improving the technique of **microinjection** of **spermatozoa** directly into eggs

Risks of Harm

In all research, the value of the knowledge to be gained must be balanced with the risk of harm that is incurred. In the case of preembryo research, there are 3 areas of potential harm. First, some preembryo research, such as in vitro testing and genetic therapy, can be scientifically validated and clinically beneficial only if there is subsequent transfer of the preembryo to a woman's uterus in an attempt to achieve pregnancy. Although such research may enhance the prospects for a normal, successful pregnancy, it also may reduce them. Second, preembryo research may be performed in a way that risks infringement of the rights of sperm and **oocyte** donors. Third, the harm that is of central concern to many, however, is the potential harm to the preembryo itself—not only damage but sometimes destruction, and the possible subjection of the preembryo to research that is not aimed at its own benefit. Allied to this is a concern that the manipulation of preembryos will diminish societal respect for human life in general. It is this third area of potential harms that has motivated the attention of national ethics advisory committees and commissions to the question of the moral status of the preembryo. As more and more biologic information has become available, it has shaped judgments regarding the degree of moral weight to be given to a preembryo. Because this information is relevant to many of the ethical questions surrounding preembryo research, it is useful to begin with the knowledge available about the biologic processes involved (as of 1994).

Fertilization and Preembryonic Development Stages

The process out of which a human preembryo emerges is complex (Fig. 2) (7–11). The scientific description of this process uses terms that are morally neutral and extremely helpful for identifying the biologic entity with which this chapter is concerned. Thus, for example, the preembryo refers to an entity in a stage of development that begins after fertilization and ends approximately 14 days later with the appearance of the **primitive streak** (that is, the band of cells at the caudal end of the **embryonic disc** from which the **embryo** develops). The characteristics of the preembryo, insofar as they are known, are understandable only within the details of the process that precedes the preembryo and the process of which it is itself a part. Hence, it is necessary to add some details to the description of fertilization and the early development that follows fertilization.

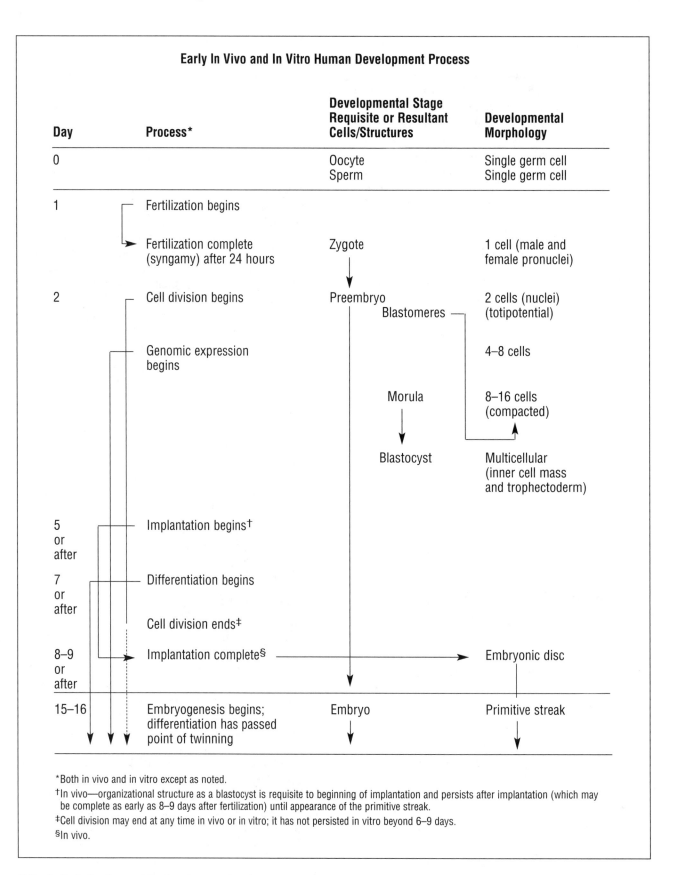

FIG. 2. Early in vivo and in vitro human development process.

Fertilization

Fertilization is a complex biochemical process and sequence of events that takes approximately 24 hours after penetration of the oocyte by the sperm (12). It usually occurs in the fallopian tube at the end nearest the ovary. It begins with contact of the male and female gametes, continues with the gradual penetration of the sperm into the various layers of the oocyte, and is completed when the **pronuclei** of the sperm and oocyte lose their nuclear membranes and fuse to form a new cell called the **zygote**. Paternal and maternal genetic contributions during the fertilization process are from separate pronuclei; as separate entities, they can be experimentally removed from the process. The last stage of the mingling process is called **syngamy**. In this stage, the male and female **haploid** chromosome sets finally fuse, following the breakdown of their pronuclear membranes, into a zygote, a **diploid** cell with 46 chromosomes.

Early Preembryonic Development

After syngamy, the zygote undergoes mitotic cell division as it moves down the fallopian tube toward the uterus. The first division takes approximately 20 hours. A series of mitotic divisions then leads to the development of the preembryo. The newly divided cells are called **blastomeres**. From 1 to 3 days after syngamy, there is a division into 2 cells, then 4 cells. Approximately 3 days after syngamy, the developing entity reaches the 8-cell stage, and from 4 to 5 days, the 8-cell to 16-cell stages. Blastomeres form cellular aggregates of distinct, **totipotent**, undifferentiated cells that, during several early cell divisions, retain the capacity to develop independently into normal preembryos. Single blastomeres are distinct until after the 8-cell to 16-cell stages when changes occur in their membranes and cytoplasms that allow them to adhere more tightly to one another during the process of compaction to form the **morula**.

Several interesting observations can be made about the earliest stages of cell division. For example, with the first 3 and possibly 4 cell divisions (during the first 1–4 days after syngamy), there is no fusion between the individual cells. What exists is a loose collection of distinct totipotent cells (blastomeres) held together by the zona pellucida. Therefore, there is as yet no designation of an individual cell to become a specific entity or a particular part of an entity. In addition, early events such as chromosomal condensation and pronuclear formation may be controlled by factors within the oocyte cytoplasm before fertilization. Messenger RNA

from the oocyte, along with oocyte organelles, supports the nutritional, synthetic, and energetic requirements of the preembryo. The function of the new genes of the preembryo cannot be detected until the 4-cell to 8-cell stage, even though the 46 chromosomes of the developing entity (23 from the oocyte and 23 from the sperm) have associated at syngamy. Experimental evidence suggests that expression of the paternal genome does occur approximately during the 8-cell stage (13, 14). Thus, the single-cell and 2-cell stages of human development appear to be regulated by information derived from the oocyte (not from the fused gametes). Activation of gene function of the preembryo first occurs between the 4-cell and 8-cell stages of development (36–72 hours after fertilization). Also, although the number of cells of the developing entity increases from 2 to 4 to 8, and so forth, the blastomeres produced at each cycle of division become progressively smaller; the size of the preembryo does not therefore increase at these stages. It remains essentially the size of the fertilized oocyte.

From 4 to 5 days after syngamy, the compacted morula develops into a **blastocyst**, which is a cellular aggregate with a central cavity, a **trophectoderm**, and a distinct **inner cell mass**. The multicellular blastocyst, now within the uterus, remains unattached in the uterine cavity fluid for approximately 48 hours. After this (now 5–7 days after syngamy), the process of implantation begins.

Implantation

As the blastocyst is in the process of attaching to the uterine wall, the cells increase in number and organize into 2 layers of cells. Implantation progresses as the outer cell layer of the blastocyst, the trophectoderm, invades the uterine wall and erodes blood vessels and glands. Having begun 5 or more days after fertilization with the attachment of the blastocyst to the endometrial lining of the uterus, implantation is completed when the blastocyst is fully embedded in the endometrium several days later. The extraembryonic outer cell layer establishes a complex interaction with maternal uterine tissues to allow implantation to continue, and these cells give rise to the placenta and membranes. The inner cell mass is the progenitor of all the cells and cell types of the future embryo. But, at this time, these cells are not yet totally differentiated in terms of their determination to specific cells or organs of the embryo.

The term preembryo, then, includes the developmental stages from the first cell division of the zygote through the morula and the blastocyst. By approximately the 14th day after the end of the process of fertilization, all cells, depending on their position, will have become parts of the placenta and membranes or the embryo. The "embryo" stage, therefore, begins approximately 16 days after the beginning of the fertilization process and continues until the end of 8 weeks after fertilization, when organogenesis is complete.

Ethical Relevance of Scientific Information

Scientific information alone cannot resolve questions about the moral status of the preembryo. Scientists themselves sometimes disagree in interpreting available data, and science is not the sole arbiter in debates about values. Nonetheless, embedded in scientific descriptions of the processes of preembryonic development are at least 2 factors that may influence the evaluation of the moral status of the preembryo—and, hence, the ethical arguments concerning preembryo research. These 2 factors, taken into account by national committees and commissions that have identified a 14-day limit for research on human preembryos, are 1) the lack of individuation of the developing entity during that period and 2) the natural failure of a high percentage of zygotes to develop into embryos.

Individuation or Singleness

From what is known about developing preembryos, their final individuation as entities with a concrete potential to become human persons is only accomplished with development of the primitive streak approximately 14 days after the completion of the fertilization process (15–17). Several factors are relevant to this observation. First, fertilization is not a momentary event but a 2-day process. Second, once fertilization is completed, there is an entity with a new genotype. But this entity is not, at its earliest stages, capable of expression (ie, **transcription**) of the new genotype, being regulated instead by information from the oocyte for continued growth and development. Third, relevant animal research has demonstrated that in the initial stages of preembryonic development a) up to at least the 8-cell stage, 1 or more blastomeres can be removed from the aggregate and the remainder can still produce a complete adult; b) individual blastomeres can be removed and develop into a complete individual; and c) cells derived from 2 preembryos of different genetic origin can aggregate into one larger mass and develop into one individual called a **chimera**. Fourth, and

perhaps most notable, from the earliest stages of cell division all the way to the complete formation of the primitive streak, the preembryo is capable of dividing into more than 1 entity. Twinning may occur during the development of the inner cell mass, or, even later, the primitive streak may split and form 2 centers that organize the development of separate preembryos. Such splits and separations may be incomplete, resulting in the formation of conjoined twins. Hence, division and recombination may occur up to 14 days after fertilization. Only after this period has **differentiation** of embryonic cells advanced to the point that separation can no longer result in 2 or more individuals.

The evidence that there is, for approximately 14 days after fertilization is complete, not yet an individuated human entity determined for development as a single being is arguably relevant to an assessment of the moral status of the preembryo. It can yield a conclusion that the human preembryo does not possess the biologic individuality necessary for a concrete potentiality to become a human person, even though it does possess a unique human genotype. The preembryo can thus be considered valuable but not at the same level as a human person.

Spontaneous Early Preembryo Loss

Not unrelated to the issue of lack of individuation is the evidence that there is a naturally high percentage of loss of preembryos. That is, in unassisted human reproduction, the development and spontaneous loss of preembryos is a frequent occurrence (18–21). Traditionally, the generally accepted findings have been that 10–15% of clinically recognized pregnancies terminate in spontaneous abortion. Data based on the use of highly sensitive assays for human chorionic gonadotropin indicate that a significant number of losses occur subclinically. Research has shown that up to 60% of fertilizations do not survive long enough to result in a missed menstrual period. Approximately one half of chemically detected pregnancies are lost during the first postovulatory week. This high rate of early losses may be caused by errors in gametogenesis, defects in the fertilization process, developmental abnormalities after fertilization, or a delay in implantation secondary to altered tubal transport time. Whatever the reasons, natural reproduction occurs in such a way that more than one half (some estimates range as high as 78%) of fertilizations do not result in live births. According to available data, in vivo pregnancy loss is highest in the first 14 days after fertilization, precisely the same developmental period in which in vitro preembryo research would be taking place.

Successful fertilization and early cell division stages of the preembryo require a complex biochemical environment that can be artificially provided in the laboratory for some species. Investigators have not sustained viable in vitro human preembryos beyond 6–9 days after fertilization. Up to the point at which the in vitro human preembryo ceases to demonstrate cell division, the developmental changes that occur and the chances of loss are similar to those during in vivo development.

The high rate of loss of preembryos during in vivo development may undergird the conclusion that the moral status of preembryos is to be differentiated from that of embryos. The ACOG Committee on Ethics notes this, although it regards considerations of lack of settled individuality in the preembryo as a more significant basis for this conclusion.

Ethical Considerations

The context for the ethical recommendations and commentary that follow is the clinical situation in which prospective parents seek assistance in their goals of pregnancy and childbearing. In this context of treatment for infertility, some preembryos not ultimately dedicated to the goal of pregnancy may become available for research. Although generated for procreation, they become "spare" preembryos, and they may then (through their use in research) serve a secondary purpose of overcoming human problems of procreation in general.

The ethical question of whether preembryos should be generated solely for the purpose of scientific research is not explicitly addressed by these guidelines. Without the further ethical analysis required to evaluate this possibility, the Committee on Ethics takes only the position that it is preferable to use spare preembryos rather than to generate preembryos specifically for research. The reasons for this position include a concern not to place women at unnecessary risk during the required ovulation induction process and a preference for a process that is less vulnerable to the commercialization of gametes.

Guidelines

The Committee on Ethics recommends the following guidelines for clinical and laboratory research on the preembryo. Some of these guidelines parallel general ethical guidelines for research on human

subjects (22), but some are particular to the case of research on human preembryos.

Research on the human preembryo may be conducted under the following conditions:

1. Research is conducted only by scientifically qualified individuals and in settings that include appropriate and adequate resources and protections.
2. The question to be explored is scientifically valid in the sense that it takes into account scientific work to date.
3. The information sought offers potential scientific and clinical benefit relative to the growth and development of the preembryo or embryo.
4. The research objectives cannot be met through research on animals or on nonfertilized gametes.
5. The design of the research and each of its procedures is clearly formulated in a research protocol that is submitted to a specially appointed independent committee, such as an institutional review board, for evaluation, guidance, and approval. The protocol includes provision for detailed records of the study.
6. The research will be concluded at the earliest possible developmental stage of the preembryo.
7. Any preembryo that has undergone research will be transferred to a uterus only if the research was related to the preembryo's preparation for placement and there is reasonable scientific confidence in its normal development.
8. The research protocol does not involve the purchase or sale of preembryos.
9. Potential donors of gametes are adequately informed of the goals, methods, anticipated benefits, and potential hazards of research. Each potential donor is informed that she or he is at liberty to refuse participation in the research and to withdraw from the research.
10. Gamete donors are provided with the opportunity to determine, with adequate information and freedom, the disposition of preembryos. This presupposes an explicit policy on the part of the researchers and their sponsoring institutions—a policy that articulates options and that provides for informed donor choice.

Ethical Commentary on Guidelines

Because some of the guidelines express standard ethical and scientific requirements for research, they need no comment. Others, however, call for further clarification or support. Underlying all of the guidelines is the ethical position that if preembryo research is to be justifiable, it must be guided by a particular application of ethical standards parallel to those for research on human subjects. This position itself can now be more clearly focused along with clarifications of particular guidelines.

Guideline 4: Creating a Preliminary Knowledge Base for Human Research. Guideline 4 expresses the reasonable ethical maxim that human research should be engaged in only when alternative means of developing knowledge are inadequate. Whenever possible, animal models or cell and tissue culture systems should be used to advance the understanding of human biology. However, direct extrapolation of results from in vitro animal preembryo studies to humans can be misleading. Unfertilized oocytes also do not offer the same opportunities for knowledge of growth processes as do preembryos.

Guidelines 6–8: Limits to Preembryo Research. The Committee on Ethics takes the position that human preembryo research can be justified under certain conditions. This position is based on an interpretation of the moral status of the preembryo as a living entity with a human genetic code, deserving of some form of respect in itself and not solely for its usefulness in research. But this position also recognizes the value of the preembryo as relative, in the sense that it does not require the degree of protection and absolute respect that is accorded to human persons. In other words, the preembryo is human—not simply like other human tissue (for it is genetically unique and has human potential), but it also is not a human person and does not as yet have within itself a determinate potential to become an individual human person (it lacks settled unity and individuality, and it evidences a high level of natural loss before implantation). On this interpretation, risks of harm to the preembryo in research can be justified, but not without limits. Preembryos, for example, should not be subjected to frivolous or poorly designed research programs; each succeeding developmental stage requires stronger justifications for doing research involving risk of harm; if the preembryos are designated for transfer to a uterus, the goals of successful pregnancy are given priority; and the real and symbolic values of the preembryo are not negated or trivialized by treating them as commodities.

Guidelines 9–10: Donation and Consent. Although informed consent of participants is a basic requirement in all human research, particular issues in decisions about preembryo research deserve elaboration. Among the most urgent of these issues is what to do with those preembryos that are not transferred to a uterus or are transferred only after research or a storage interval.

To enhance the probability that adequate numbers of normally developing preembryos will result, more oocytes usually are fertilized in vitro than will be transferred to the woman. If the number of resulting normally developing preembryos exceeds expectations, questions arise regarding the disposition of unused preembryos. Possible options may include **cryopreservation** of preembryos for the couple's future use, donation of preembryos to a recipient who is unable to produce usable oocytes or whose genetic background makes it inadvisable for her to use her own oocytes, donation of preembryos for research, and disposal of preembryos.

The appropriate individuals to exercise responsible decision making regarding the disposition of preembryos are the individuals who provide the gametes. Their informed consent is required before preembryos are used in research. The gamete donors in IVF should presumptively have an equal say in the use of their preembryos; therefore, the preembryos should not be used for research without the consent of both parties. If research is to be done on a preembryo that is to be transferred to a third party, this individual and the individuals who plan to rear the potential child (if different from the gamete donors) also should give informed consent.

Each IVF program should develop policies regarding the options of transfer, storage, donation, research, and discard. These policies should cover the disposition of gametes and of both normally developing preembryos and preembryos with a preimplantation diagnosis of genetic disease. They should include provision for counseling gamete providers and for fullest possible implementation of informed consent. Policies should be developed in light of ethical and legal considerations, and they should cover eventualities such as informing gamete providers of what will be done with preembryos in the absence of a written statement of the gamete providers' wishes.

Couples considering IVF therapy should be fully informed of the options available to them and of the policies of the IVF program. Their choices should be made in circumstances free of financial or other coercion. Full information should therefore include assurance that consent to donation of preembryos for research is not a condition for receiving services and that fee scales are not contingent on consent to research. Gamete providers also should be made aware of the possible need for further choices in the future (eg, when cryopreservation is involved, passing time may alter circumstances and affect choices).

Conclusion

The Committee on Ethics has offered a position that approves preembryo research but limits it according to ethical guidelines. This position advocates treatment of the preembryo with respect but not the same level of respect as is given to human persons. It is a position that will be acceptable even to those who accord full respect to embryos and fetuses but not to those who believe that full respect should be extended to the gamete, zygote, and preembryo throughout the process of fertilization and beyond. In arriving at its position, the Committee on Ethics considered scientific and clinical information relevant to ethical analysis, although it recognizes the role of both scientific and ethical interpretation of what cannot be simply incontrovertible "facts."

The Committee on Ethics once again acknowledges that no single position can encompass the variety of opinions within the membership of ACOG, and it affirms that no physician should be required to participate in preembryo research if he or she finds it morally objectionable. Nonetheless, it is important to public discourse and to the practice of responsible medicine that physicians become aware of the medical and ethical issues involved in the complex area of preembryo research. To advance this discourse, it is helpful for physicians to reflect on and share the basis of their own views and to recognize and explore the ethical perspectives of their patients and colleagues.

Glossary

Blastocyst: A stage in early human development that follows from the formation of the morula. The blastocyst is a sphere of cells containing a fluid-filled cavity forming approximately 4 days after fertilization and before the beginning of the process of implantation.

Blastomeres: The cells derived from the first and subsequent cell divisions of the zygote.

Chimera: An organism composed of cells derived from an aggregation of cells originating from 2 different genotypes. Such an aggregation is possible up to the 8-cell stage.

Cryopreservation: Storage by freezing.

Differentiation: The process of acquiring individual characteristics, as occurs in progressive diversification of cells and tissues of the developing preembryo and embryo.

Diploid: A cell having 2 chromosome sets, usually one maternal and one paternal, twice the haploid number (in humans, 46).

Donors: Individuals providing either sperm or ova.

Embryo: The stage in human development starting from approximately 2 weeks after fertilization, with organization around a single primitive streak, and continuing until the end of the eighth week after fertilization when all major structures are represented.

Embryonic disc: The group of cells from which the embryo will develop, usually visible at the end of the first week of development after fertilization in humans.

Fertilization: The process which renders gametes capable of further development; it begins when the sperm contacts the plasma membrane of the oocyte and ends with the formation of the zygote.

Gametes: Mature reproductive cells, usually haploid in chromosome number (eg, sperm or ovum).

Haploid: The chromosome number of a normal gamete (sperm or ovum). In humans, the haploid number is 23, representing 1 member of each chromosome pair.

Implantation: Attachment of the blastocyst to the endometrial lining of the uterus and subsequent embedding in the endometrium. Implantation begins approximately 5–7 days after fertilization and may be complete as early as 8–9 days after fertilization.

Inner cell mass: The centrally located cells within the blastocyst; these cells will develop into the embryo.

Microinjection (of sperm): Injection of 1 or more sperm under the outer covering of the oocyte for fertilization.

Morula: A compact sphere of 16 blastomeres that forms approximately 3–4 days after fertilization.

Oocyte: An immature female reproductive cell, one that has not completed the maturing process to form an ovum (gamete).

Preembryo: The developing cells produced by the division of the zygote until the formation of the embryo proper at the appearance of the primitive streak approximately 14 days after fertilization.

Primitive streak: The initial band of cells from which the embryo begins to develop, located at the caudal end of the embryonic disc. The primitive streak is present approximately 15 days after fertilization.

Pronuclei: The egg and sperm nuclei after penetration of the sperm into the egg during fertilization.

Spermatozoa: Mature male germ cells (gametes).

Syngamy: The final stage of the fertilization process in which the haploid chromosome sets from the male and female gametes come together following breakdown of the pronuclear membranes to form the zygote.

Totipotent: Able to differentiate along any line; the capacity of a cell or group of cells to produce all of the products of conception—the extra-embryonic membrane and tissue, the embryo, and, subsequently, the fetus.

Transcription: Transfer of genetic code information from one kind of nucleic acid to another.

Trophectoderm: Peripheral cells of the blastocyst that form the membrane sac surrounding the embryo.

Zygote: The single cell formed by the union of the male and female haploid gametes at syngamy.

References

1. Research involving pregnant women or fetuses. 45 C.F.R. §46.204 (2002).
2. U.S. Department of Health, Education, and Welfare. HEW support of research involving human in vitro fertilization and embryo transfer. Washington, DC: U.S. Government Printing Office; 1979.
3. Research on preembryos: justifications and limitations. American Fertility Society. Fertil Steril 1986;46(3 Suppl):56S–57S.
4. Research on preembryos: justifications and limitations. American Fertility Society. Fertil Steril 1990;53(Suppl 2):62S–63S.
5. The Committee to Consider the Social, Ethical and Legal Issues Arising from In Vitro Fertilization (Victoria). Report on the disposition of embryos produced by in vitro fertilization. Melbourne (AUS): The Committee; 1984.
6. Department of Health and Social Security (UK). Scientific issues. In: Report of the Committee on Inquiry into Human Fertilisation and Embryology. London: Her Majesty's Stationery Office; 1984. p. 58–69.
7. Kalousek DK, Lau AE, Baldwin VJ. Development of the embryo, fetus, and placenta. In: Dimmick JE, Kalousek DK, editors. Developmental pathology of the embryo and fetus. Philadelphia (PA): JB Lippincott; 1992. p. 1–25.
8. Moore KL, Persaud TV. The developing human: clinically oriented embryology. 7th ed. Philadelphia (PA): Saunders; 2003.
9. Sadler TW. First week of development: ovulation to implantation. In: Langman's medical embryology. 9th ed. Philadelphia (PA): Lippincott Williams & Wilkins; 2004. p. 31–49.
10. Jones HW Jr, Schrader C. And just what is a pre-embryo? Fertil Steril 1989;52:189–91.
11. Grobstein C. The early development of human embryos. J Med Philos 1985;10:213–36.
12. Veeck LL. Fertilization and early embryonic development. Curr Opin Obstet Gynecol 1992;4:702–11.
13. Braude P, Bolton V, Moore S. Human gene expression first occurs between the four- and eight-cell stages of preimplantation development. Nature 1988;332:459–61.
14. O'Farrell PH, Edgar BA, Lakich D, Lehner CF. Directing cell division during development. Science 1989;246:635–40.
15. McCormick RA. Who or what is the preembryo? Kennedy Inst Ethics J 1991;1:1–15.
16. Grobstein C. Becoming an individual. In: Science and the unborn. New York (NY): Basic Books; 1988. p. 21–39.
17. Ethical considerations of the new reproductive technologies: III. Considerations on the status of human gametes and preembryos. Society of Obstetricians and Gynaecologists of Canada. J SOGC 1992;14(6):84–5.
18. Chard T. Frequency of implantation and early pregnancy loss in natural cycles. Baillières Clin Obstet Gynecol 1991;5:179–89.
19. Wilcox AJ, Weinberg CR, Wehmann RE, Armstrong EG, Canfield RE, Nisula BC. Measuring early pregnancy loss: laboratory and field methods. Fertil Steril 1985;44:366–74.
20. Wilcox AJ, Weinberg CR, O'Connor JF, Baird DD, Schlatterer JP, Canfield RE, et al. Incidence of early loss of pregnancy. N Engl J Med 1988;319:189–94.
21. Edmonds DK, Lindsay KS, Miller JF, Williamson E, Wood PJ. Early embryonic mortality in women. Fertil Steril 1982;38:447–53.
22. Beauchamp TL, Walters L, editors. Contemporary issues in bioethics. 6th ed. Belmont (CA): Wadsworth; 2003.

Bibliography

The Committee to Consider the Social, Ethical and Legal Issues Arising from In Vitro Fertilization (Victoria). Report on the disposition of embryos produced by in vitro fertilization. Melbourne (AUS): The Committee; 1984.

Department of Health and Social Security (UK). Scientific issues. In: Report of the Committee on Inquiry into Human Fertilisation and Embryology. London: Her Majesty's Stationery Office; 1984. p. 58–69.

Grobstein C. Science and the unborn. New York (NY): Basic Books; 1988.

Protection of human subjects. 45 C.F.R. Part 46 (2002).

Research on preembryos: justifications and limitations. American Fertility Society. Fertil Steril 1990;53(Suppl 2): 62S–63S.

Seppälä M, editor. Factors of importance for implantation. Baillières Clin Obstet Gynaecol 1991;5:1–252.

Singer P, Kuhse H, Buckle S, Dawson K, Kasimba P, editors. Embryo experimentation. New York (NY): Cambridge University Press; 1990.

U.S. Department of Health, Education, and Welfare. HEW support of research involving human in vitro fertilization and embryo transfer. Washington, DC: U.S. Government Printing Office; 1979.

Walters L. Ethics and new reproductive technologies: an international review of committee statements. Hastings Cent Rep 1987;17(3):S3–9.

Suggested Reading

American Academy of Pediatrics. Committee on Pediatric Research and Committee on Bioethics. Human embryo research [Published erratum appears in Pediatrics 2001;108:1221]. Pediatrics 2001;108:813–6.

The biologic characteristics of the preembryo. American Fertility Society. Fertil Steril 1994;62(5 suppl):29S–31S.

Informed consent and the use of gametes and embryos for research. The Ethics Committee of the American Society for Reproductive Medicine. Fertil Steril 1997;68:780–1.

The moral and legal status of the preembryo. American Fertility Society. Fertil Steril 1994;62(5 suppl):32S–34S.

National Bioethics Advisory Commission. Ethical issues in human stem cell research. Volume I: report and recommendations on the National Bioethics Advisory Commission. Rockville (MD): NBAC; 1999.

Research on preembryos: justifications and limitations. American Fertility Society. Fertil Steril 1994;62(5 suppl): 78S–80S.

Sexual Misconduct

The privilege of caring for patients, often over a long period, can yield considerable professional satisfaction. The obstetrician–gynecologist may fill many roles for patients, including primary physician, technology expert, prevention specialist, counselor, and confidante. Privy to both birth and death, obstetrician–gynecologists assist women as they pass through adolescence; grow into maturity; make choices about sexuality, partnership, and family; experience the sorrows of reproductive loss, infertility, and illness; and adapt to the transitions of midlife and aging. The practice of obstetrics and gynecology includes interaction at times of intense emotion and vulnerability for the patient and involves both sensitive physical examinations and medically necessary disclosure of especially private information about symptoms and experiences. The relationship between the physician and patient, therefore, requires a high level of trust and professional responsibility.

Trust of this sort cannot be maintained without a basic understanding of the limits and responsibilities of the professional's role. Physician sexual misconduct is an example of abuse of limits and failure of responsibility. The valued human experience of the physician–patient relationship is damaged when there is either confusion regarding professional goals and behavior or clear lack of integrity that allows sexual exploitation and harm.

Sexual misconduct is of particular concern in today's environment of shifting roles for women and men, greater sexual freedom, and critical evaluation of power relations in society (1–4). Prohibitions against sexual contact between patient and physician are not new, however; they can be found in the earliest guidelines in western antiquity. From the beginning, physicians were enjoined to "do no harm" and specifically avoid sexual contact with patients (5). In

the intervening centuries, as the study of medical ethics has evolved, attention has been focused on respect for individual rights, the problem of unequal power in relationships between professionals and patients, and the potential for abuse of that power (6).

In this context, the American Medical Association's Council on Ethical and Judicial Affairs developed a report, "Sexual Misconduct in the Practice of Medicine," condemning sexual relations between physicians and current patients (7). It raises serious questions about the ethics of romantic relationships with former patients. It is summarized as follows:

> Sexual contact that occurs concurrent with the physician–patient relationship constitutes sexual misconduct. Sexual or romantic interactions between physicians and patients detract from the goals of the physician–patient relationship, may exploit the vulnerability of the patient, may obscure the physician's objective judgment concerning the patient's health care, and ultimately may be detrimental to the patient's well-being (8).

The Council provides the following clear guidelines (7):

- Mere mutual consent is rejected as a justification for sexual relations with patients because the disparity in power, status, vulnerability, and need make it difficult for a patient to give meaningful consent to sexual contact or sexual relations.

- Sexual contact or a romantic relationship concurrent with the physician–patient relationship is unethical.

- Sexual contact or a romantic relationship with a former patient may be unethical under certain circumstances. The relevant standard is the potential for misuse of physician power and exploitation of

Previously published as Committee Opinion 144, November 1994

patient emotions derived from the former relationship.

- Education on ethical issues involved in sexual misconduct should be included throughout all levels of medical training.
- Physicians have a responsibility to report offending colleagues to disciplinary boards.

The Society of Obstetricians and Gynaecologists of Canada has adopted a similar statement that "acknowledges and deplores the fact that incidents of physicians abusing patients do occur" and finds that "these incidents include 'sexual impropriety' due to poor clinical skills, chauvinism, or abuse of the power relationship, and outright systematic sexual abuse" (9). The Society also supports the right to "informed, safe, and gender-sensitive" care and the right of victims of abuse to receive "prompt treatment." "Identification, discipline, and, where possible, rehabilitation of the perpetrators" is recommended.

Although much discussion of sexual misconduct by physicians in the past decade has centered around the particular vulnerability that exists within the psychiatrist–patient relationship (10), sexual contact between patients and obstetrician–gynecologists also has been documented. Physicians themselves acknowledge that there is a problem, but the extent of the problem is difficult to determine because information relies on self-reporting, which carries the potential for bias in response.

The Committee on Ethics of the American College of Obstetricians and Gynecologists endorses the ethical principles expressed by the American Medical Association and the Society of Obstetricians and Gynaecologists of Canada and affirms the following statements:

- Sexual contact or a romantic relationship between a physician and a current patient is always unethical.
- Sexual contact or a romantic relationship between a physician and a former patient also may be unethical. Potential risks to both parties should be considered carefully. Such risks may stem from length of time and intensity of the previous professional relationship; age differences; the length of time since cessation of the professional relationship; the former patient's residual feelings of dependency, obligation, or gratitude; the patient's vulnerability to manipulation as a result of private information disclosed during treatment; or physician vulnerability if a relationship initiated with a former patient breaks down.

- Physicians should be careful not to mix roles that are ordinarily in conflict. For example, they should not perform breast or pelvic examinations on their own minor children unless an urgent indication exists. Children and adolescents are particularly vulnerable to emotional conflict and damage to their developing sense of identity and sexuality when roles and role boundaries with trusted adults are confused. It is essential to ensure the young individual's privacy and prevent subtly coercive violations from occurring.
- The request by either a patient or a physician to have a chaperon present during a physical examination should be accommodated irrespective of the physician's sex. Local practices and expectations differ with regard to the use of chaperons, but the presence of a third party in the examination room can confer benefits for both patient and physician, regardless of the sex of the chaperon. Chaperons can provide reassurance to the patient about the professional context and content of the examination and the intention of the physician and offer witness to the actual events taking place should there be any misunderstanding. The presence of a third party in the room may, however, cause some embarrassment to the patient and limit her willingness to talk openly with the physician because of concerns about confidentiality. If a chaperon is present, the physician should provide a separate opportunity for private conversation. If the chaperon is an employee of the practice, the physician must establish clear rules about respect for privacy and confidentiality. In addition, some patients (especially, but not limited to, adolescents) may consider the presence of a family member as an intrusion. Family members should not be used as chaperons unless specifically requested by the patient.
- Examinations should be performed with only the necessary amount of physical contact required to obtain data for diagnosis and treatment. Appropriate explanation should accompany all examination procedures.
- Physicians should avoid sexual innuendo and sexually provocative remarks.
- When physicians have questions and concerns about their sexual feelings and behavior, they should seek advice from mentors or appropriate professional organizations (11).
- It is important for physicians to self-monitor for any early indications that the barrier between normal sexual feelings and inappropriate behavior is

not being maintained (12). These indicators might include special scheduling, seeing a patient outside of normal office hours or outside the office, driving a patient home, or making sexually explicit comments about patients.

- Physicians involved in medical education should actively work to include as part of the basic curriculum information about both physician and patient vulnerability, avoidance of sexually offensive or denigrating language, risk factors for sexual misconduct, and procedures for reporting and rehabilitation.

- Physicians aware of instances of sexual misconduct on the part of any health professional have an obligation to report such situations to appropriate authorities, such as institutional committee chairs, department chairs, peer review organizations, supervisors, or professional licensing boards.

- Physicians with administrative responsibilities in hospitals, other medical institutions, and licensing boards should develop clear and public guidelines for reporting instances of sexual misconduct, prompt investigation of all complaints, and appropriate disciplinary and remedial action.

In conclusion, sexual misconduct on the part of physicians is an abuse of professional power and a violation of patient trust. It jeopardizes the well-being of patients and carries an immense potential for harm. The ethical prohibition against physician sexual misconduct is ancient and forceful, and its application to contemporary medical practice is essential.

References

1. Kardener SH, Fuller M, Mensh IN. A survey of physicians' attitudes and practices regarding erotic and nonerotic contact with patients. Am J Psychiatry 1973;130:1077–81.

2. Wilbers D, Veenstra G, van de Wiel HB, Schultz WC. Sexual contact in the doctor–patient relationship in The Netherlands. BMJ 1992;304:1531–4.

3. Gartrell NK, Milliken N, Goodson WH 3rd, Thiemann S, Lo B. Physician–patient sexual contact. Prevalence and problems. West J Med 1992;157:139–43.

4. Johnson SH. Judicial review of disciplinary action for sexual misconduct in the practice of medicine. JAMA 1993;270:1596–600.

5. Campbell ML. The oath: an investigation of the injunction prohibiting physician–patient sexual relations. Perspect Biol Med 1989;32:300–8.

6. Beauchamp TL, Childress JF. Principles of biomedical ethics. 5th ed. New York (NY): Oxford University Press; 2001.

7. Sexual misconduct in the practice of medicine. American Medical Association, Council on Ethical and Judicial Affairs. JAMA 1991;266:2741–5.

8. Sexual misconduct in the practice of medicine. American Medical Association, Council on Ethical and Judicial Affairs. Code of medical ethics: current opinions with annotations. Chicago (IL): AMA; 2002. p. 230–3.

9. Sexual abuse by physicians. SOGC Policy Statement No. 134. Society of Obstetricians and Gynaecologists of Canada. J Obstet Gynaecol Can 2003;25:862.

10. Gabbard GO, editor. Sexual exploitation in professional relationships. Washington, DC: American Psychiatric Press; 1989.

11. Abel GG, Barrett DH, Gardos PS. Sexual misconduct by physicians. J Med Assoc Ga 1992;81:237–46.

12. Searight HR, Campbell DC. Physician–patient sexual contact: ethical and legal issues and clinical guidelines. J Fam Pract 1993;36:647–53.

PART IV
Societal Responsibilities

"A physician shall recognize a responsibility to participate in activities contributing to the improvement of the community and the betterment of public health."—American Medical Association, "Principles of Medical Ethics"

Care rendered to an individual patient does not take place in a vacuum but rather within a community. Decisions made in one sphere affect those in the other. Obstetrician–gynecologists have a responsibility not only to their individual patients but also to society as a whole. Accordingly, they should support and participate in activities that enhance the community. These activities may include the organization, administration, and evaluation of the health care system; public health activities; consultation with and advice to community leaders, government officials, and members of the judiciary; or expert witness testimony.

In this part of Ethics in Obstetrics and Gynecology, *the ethical issues associated with conflict of interest take on special importance. Different segments of society stand to benefit in different ways from an obstetrician–gynecologist's actions, and finding a proper balance can be challenging. These chapters outline ethical approaches to several situations that may be faced by obstetrician–gynecologists as they seek to fulfill their responsibilities to society.*

Relationships With Industry

Manufacturers of pharmaceuticals and medical devices assist physicians in the pursuit of their educational goals and objectives through financial support of various medical, research, and educational programs. Industrial development of products is important to continuing improvement in health care.

Corporations are primarily responsible to their stockholders, while physicians are primarily responsible to their patients. The goals of corporations may conflict with physicians' duties to their patients.

In the past, physicians and their professional organizations often have uncritically accepted gifts from pharmaceutical corporations in the belief that such gifts did not necessarily create undue influence on medical practice. Evidence has accumulated, however, about the extent to which gifts from industry may misdirect physicians from their primary responsibility, which is to act consistently in the best interests of their patients. Studies demonstrate that the prescribing practices of physicians are commonly influenced by both subtle and obvious marketing messages and gifts, even when delivered in an educational context, and even when the physicians studied did not recognize or admit to any changes in their practice of medicine (1).

When members of industry interact with the American College of Obstetricians and Gynecologists and its Fellows, corporate activities may generate biases or obligations unrelated to product merit, creating the actuality or the appearance of inappropriate and undue interest on the part of physicians or organizations. The possible scope of such conflict of interest is great. In 2002, pharmaceutical companies spent $11.5 billion to provide physicians with free samples (2). This is likely to have an impact on treatment practices that is not necessarily related to the merit of the product. Biomedical research expenditures by industry exceed those of the federal government.

The public expects physicians to avoid conflicts of interest in decisions about patient care. Such decisions usually involve the direct treatment of patients. They also may involve physician participation in purchasing decisions by medical organizations, such as hospitals and group practices, to which physicians owe fiduciary responsibility. When any product promotion or research project leads to inappropriate or unbalanced medical advice to patients, an ethical problem exists. Sponsorship of medical activities by industrial companies and by other agencies seeking to influence medical care patterns must not distort the accuracy, completeness, or balanced presentation of medical advice to patients.

Recommendations of Other Organizations

The American Medical Association (AMA) has addressed gifts to physicians from industry in the context of clinical practice and support of continuing medical education (CME) or professional meetings (3, 4). The American College of Physicians–American Society of Internal Medicine has issued guidelines both on relationships of individual physicians with industry and on relationships of organizations with industry (5, 6).

The implications of industry support on medical education have been addressed as they affect postgraduate training and CME. In 2002, the Accreditation Council for Graduate Medical Education issued guidance for the more than 7,700 residency programs in the United States (7). The Accreditation Council for Continuing Medical Education (ACCME) has issued guidelines that address the support of educational programs and the provision of related

Previously published as Committee Opinion 259, October 2001; content revised January 2004 awards, grants, and contracts (8). The ACCME guidelines are being revised. Proposed changes note that some conflicts of interest are so fundamental that they cannot be addressed adequately by disclosure and would require exclusion of the individual or firm from controlling the content of CME. These proposed revisions have been criticized as an attack on professional freedom (9). Current guidelines are available at the ACCME web site (www.accme.org).

Pharmaceutical Research and Manufacturers of America (PhRMA) has developed guidelines for the pharmaceutical industry's relationship with clinicians (10) and for conduct of clinical trials and communication of clinical trial results (11). These voluntary guidelines took effect July 1, 2002, and October 1, 2002, respectively.

In addition, guidance has been issued by the federal government. In 2003, the Office of Inspector General (OIG) at the Department of Health and Human Services issued a notice regarding voluntary compliance programs for pharmaceutical manufacturers. The guidance is intended to provide OIG's views on the fundamental elements that pharmaceutical manufacturers should consider when creating and implementing their own compliance programs and principles. Among the written policies and procedures that the OIG suggests be addressed are 1) a code of conduct and 2) potential risks, including relationships with purchasers, physicians, and sales agents (ie, gifts, entertainment, personal compensation, education grants, and research funding). The OIG guidance references the voluntary PhRMA guidelines and states "Although compliance with the PhRMA Code will not protect a manufacturer as a matter of law under the anti-kickback statue, it will substantially reduce the risk of fraud and abuse and help demonstrate a good faith effort to comply with the applicable federal health care program requirements" (12).

Recommendations of the American College of Obstetricians and Gynecologists' Committee on Ethics

Industry–physician interactions can be divided into 4 major types, as characterized in the following paragraphs. Ethical implications specific to each type of interaction also are discussed.

1. *Product promotion to individual physicians by advertising, personal communication, and provision of samples*—Physicians have an obligation to go beyond the information provided through advertising or other marketing strategies in selecting the best product for care of the patient. This includes the following measures:

   a. Physicians have an obligation to seek the most accurate sources of information about new products that they contemplate using, in addition to information provided by the products' marketers.

   b. When new products are to be used in an institutional setting, physicians should familiarize themselves with, and conform to, the relevant rules and policies of that institution.

2. *Company promotion to individual physicians and groups, including specialty societies, hospitals, and medical schools, through the support of educational activities, awards, and development contracts*—Support of educational programs and the provision of awards, grants, and contracts should follow, in principle, the guidelines of the AMA (3, 4) and the 1992 guidelines of the ACCME (8), which are adapted as follows:

   a. Any gifts accepted by an individual physician should primarily entail a benefit to patients or be related to the physician's work and should not be of substantial value. Accordingly, textbooks, modest meals, and similar gifts are appropriate if they serve a genuine educational function. Cash gifts should not be accepted.

   b. Subsidies to underwrite the costs of CME conferences or professional meetings can contribute to the improvement of patient care and, therefore, are permissible. Payments to defray the costs of a conference should not be accepted directly from the company by the physicians who are attending the conference. Funds from a commercial source should be in the form of an unrestricted educational grant made payable to the accredited sponsor for the support of programs. The ultimate decision about funding arrangements for CME activities must be the responsibility of the accredited sponsor.

   c. Subsidies from industry should not be accepted directly to pay for the costs of travel, lodging, or other personal expenses of the physicians who are attending the conferences or meetings; subsidies should not be accepted to compensate physicians for their time. Subsidies for hospitality should not be accepted apart from modest meals or social events that are held as part of a conference or meeting. Commercially supported social events at CME activities should not compete with, or take precedence over, the educational events. It is appropriate for faculty at conferences or meetings to accept reasonable honoraria and to accept reimbursement for reasonable travel, lodging, and meal expenses. It also is appropriate for consultants who provide genuine services to receive reasonable compensation and to accept reimbursement for reasonable travel, lodging, and meal expenses. Token consulting or advisory arrangements cannot be used to justify the compensation of physicians for their time or their travel, lodging, and other out-of-pocket expenses.

d. The gift of special funds to permit medical students, residents, and fellows to attend carefully selected educational conferences may be permissible as long as the selection of the students, residents, or fellows who will receive the funds is made by the academic or training institution or by the accredited CME sponsor with the full concurrence of the academic or training institution.

e. No gifts should be accepted if conditions or obligations are attached. For example, physicians should not accept gifts if they are tied to their prescribing practices. In addition, when companies underwrite medical conferences or lectures other than their own, the physicians responsible for organizing these activities should be responsible for, and control, the selection of content, faculty, educational methods, and materials.

f. Accredited CME sponsors are responsible for the content, quality, and scientific integrity of all CME activities and materials certified for credit.

g. Presentations should give a balanced view of therapeutic options. Use of generic names will contribute to this impartiality. If trade names are used, those of several companies should be used rather than only those of a single company.

h. When commercial exhibits are part of the overall program, arrangements for these should not influence the planning or interfere with the presentation of CME activities. Exhibit placement should not be a condition of support for a CME activity.

3. *Company promotion to individual physicians and groups of physicians, such as medical specialty societies, by provision of gifts, parties, trips, services, and opportunities for investment*—Such promotional practices, whether directed toward professional groups or individual physicians, must be assumed to have as their purpose the creation of attitudes or practices favorable to the donor. This may result in a real or perceived conflict of interest for the individual recipient or organization. Such ethical conflicts can interfere with patient care and may not be in keeping with the standards of professional conduct to which physicians are expected to adhere.

a. Any individual or group should carefully weigh the risks of ethical conflicts and adverse public opinion before accepting gifts, parties, trips, and services directly from industry.

b. When the obstetrician–gynecologist has a significant financial interest in or receives anything of substantial value, including royalties, from companies in the health care industry, such as a manufacturer of pharmaceuticals and medical devices, this information should be disclosed to patients and colleagues when material (see Appendix).

c. Physicians should not engage in agreements in which referral of patients to them is contingent on their use or advocacy of a product.

d. Physicians should not engage in agreements in which companies make substantial donations to a third party (eg, a hospital or a charitable organization) that is contingent on their use or advocacy of a product.

4. *Industrial sponsorship of research*—Companies must conduct clinical testing to obtain approval for the marketing of new products. This involves collaboration with physicians and clinical institutions. The following guidelines for participation in research should be followed:

a. Research trials should be conducted in accordance with the federal guidelines for the protection of human subjects (13). Investigators may presume that approval by the institutional review board of a medical school or hospital provides adequate ethical and scientific review. If the project is to be conducted in a private medical office, investigators must ascertain the nature of the ethical and scientific review process by the sponsoring corporation. If there is any question about the adequacy or efficacy of this review, investigators should seek independent consultation or submit the project to their institutions before agreeing to participate.

b. Reimbursement to investigators and their institutions for participation in research, including recruitment of subjects, should not exceed reasonable direct and indirect costs. Investigators may accept reasonable compensation for consultation or lecturing that follows participation in research.

c. Once a clinical investigator becomes involved in a research project for a company or knows that he or she might become involved, the investigator, as an individual, cannot ethically buy or sell the company's stock until the involvement ends and the results of the research are published or otherwise disseminated to the public (14).

d. The following guidelines should govern control over information gained from research (15):

- All obligations of investigators and sponsors should be contractually defined.

- Scientific freedom of independent investigators (those not employed by the funding organization) should be preserved.

- Principle investigators should be involved in decisions regarding the publication of data from their trials. Short delays in the dissemination of data generated by industry-sponsored research are acceptable to protect a patent or related proprietary interests. Prolonged delays, or suppression of information harmful to the sponsor's interests, are unethical.

- Investigators should control the use of their names in promotions.

- Project funding should not be contingent on results.

- Investigators should disclose their relationships with industry funders in publications or lectures based on the research.

In summary, industry continues to provide substantial and valuable support for physician education.

Obstetrician–gynecologists' relationships with industry should be structured in a manner that will enhance, rather than detract from, their obligations to their patients. The guidelines set forth in this chapter will contribute to this goal.

References

1. Wazana A. Physicians and the pharmaceutical industry: is a gift ever just a gift? JAMA 2000;283:373–80.
2. Kumar P, Zangg AM. IMS review: steady but not stellar. MM&M May 2003. p. 60, 62.
3. American Medical Association. Gifts to physicians from industry. In: Code of medical ethics: current opinions and annotations. Chicago (IL): AMA; 2002. p. 192–4.
4. American Medical Association. Clarification of opinion 8.061 "Gifts to physicians from industry." In: Code of medical ethics: current opinions with annotations. Chicago (IL): AMA; 2002. p. 195–203.
5. Coyle SL; Ethics and Human Rights Committee, American College of Physicians–American Society of Internal Medicine. Physician–industry relations. Part 1: individual physicians. Ann Intern Med 2002;136:396–402.
6. Coyle SL; Ethics and Human Rights Committee, American College of Physicians–American Society of Internal Medicine. Physician–industry relations. Part 2: organizational issues. Ann Intern Med 2002;136:403–6.
7. Accreditation Council for Graduate Medical Education. Principles to guide the relationship between graduate medical education and industry. Chicago (IL): ACGME; 2002. Available at http://www.acgme.org/New/GMEGuide.pdf. Retrieved July 28, 2003.
8. Accreditation Council for Continuing Medical Education. Standards for commercial support of continuing medical education. Chicago (IL): ACCME, 1992.
9. Relman AS; ACCME. Defending professional independence: ACCME's proposed new guidelines for commercial support of CME. JAMA 2003;289:2418–20.
10. Pharmaceutical Research and Manufacturers of America. PhRMA code on interactions with healthcare professionals. Washington, DC: PhRMA; 2002. Available at http://www.phrma.org/publications/policy//2002-04-19.391.pdf. Retrieved July 28, 2003.
11. PhRMA principles on conduct of clinical trials and communication of clinical trial results. Available at http://www.phrma.org/publications/policy//2002-06-24.430.pdf. Retrieved May 15, 2003.
12. Office of Inspector General, HHS. Compliance program guidance for pharmaceutical manufacturers. Fed Regist 2003;68:23731–43.
13. Protection of human subjects, 45 C.F.R. Part 46 (2002).
14. American Medical Association. Conflicts of interest: biomedical research. In: Code of medical ethics: current opinions with annotations. Chicago (IL): AMA; 2002. p. 169–70.
15. Chren MM. Independent investigators and for-profit companies. Guidelines for biomedical scientists considering funding by industry. Arch Dermatol 1994;130:432–7.

Patents, Medicine, and the Interests of Patients

New technologies and the translation of research discoveries into clinical medicine are essential for improvements in patient care. The increasing commercialization of medical discoveries, however, may hamper the dissemination of new knowledge and the ability of physicians and patients to benefit from applications of this knowledge. Many basic scientists and clinicians support the right to obtain and enforce patents on drugs, diagnostic tests, medical devices, and most recently, genes. Some primarily are concerned with recovering the costs they incur in developing new treatments and technologies. Others see patents in medicine as a legitimate means, within a society based on the principle of free enterprise, of protecting and enhancing intellectual capital.

Such patent protections may be regarded as necessary incentives for the development of new tests and treatments. They also may limit the ability of clinicians, patients, and researchers to obtain the right to use these discoveries commercially under reasonable conditions and at an affordable price. Furthermore, the issue of gene patenting poses unique challenges to knowledge development and academic collaboration because a gene sequence, unlike previous technical advances, is both a tool for pursuing scientific knowledge and the basis for any diagnostic or therapeutic application.

Patent Protections

The U.S. Patent and Trademark Office (PTO) is guided by federal statutes, regulations, and case law in granting patents. Patent protection is intended to promote research and discovery and to act as a stimulus to progress in science and the useful arts. The PTO evaluates an application for a U.S. patent to determine whether the claimed invention satisfies

Previously published jointly with the Committee on Genetics as Committee Opinion 277, November 2002

the following 3 conditions: the invention is a "new" and "useful" discovery or improvement that is "not obvious" to individuals with ordinary skill in the art (1). In evaluating patent applications, the PTO also assesses whether the specification adequately describes the invention and enables the skilled artisan to make and use it. A patent is granted for an invention that meets the 3 conditions and other requirements, such as being patentable subject matter. For example, "products of nature" can be patented if they are in an isolated form that does not occur in nature.

Patents that may affect the practice of medicine fall into 4 categories: 1) patents on medical and surgical procedures, 2) patents on surgical or diagnostic instruments, 3) patents on drugs, and 4) patents on genes and gene-based diagnostic or predictive tests. All of these types of patents raise ethical issues and may create conflicts of interest for physicians who contribute to the development of new products through research. The commercial potential of medical discoveries may motivate physicians to increase their own incomes in ways that may jeopardize the care of patients. Academic and research physicians may be offered incentives by their institutions to maximize the institution's extramural revenues through patent arrangements that restrict use by other researchers and, thus, act as barriers to further research discoveries.

Patenting Medical and Surgical Procedures

Historically, physicians have taught and shared medical information without regarding this knowledge as trade secrets to be protected from others. Physicians have a fundamental obligation to provide advice to their patients about the most appropriate care, without being influenced by any profit they might gain through associated commercial ventures. Open communication of information gained from research and experience with medical and surgical procedures is essential if safety and efficacy are to be validated or refuted by colleagues. It is through further scientific work by one's peers that diagnostic methodologies and medical procedures are either validated, refined, and improved or discarded as ineffective or unhelpful.

Some corporate or individual business arrangements—including the patenting and licensing of medical and surgical procedures—can be adverse to the welfare of patients. These arrangements present barriers to the availability of the protected procedures to other physicians and patients. Moreover, they may inhibit new research that might otherwise be stimulated by open access to information about the procedures. Investigational use of patented procedures is permitted under the "experimental use doctrine," which allows a patented invention to be used in a manner that does not interfere with the economic interests of the patent holder (ie, used with no commercial intentions).

For these reasons, the enforceability of patents covering medical and surgical procedures has been challenged, both ethically and legally. The American Medical Association asserts that it is unethical for physicians "to seek, secure or enforce patents on medical procedures" because such practices may limit the availability of new procedures to patients (2). In the 1996 case *Pallin v. Singer*, Dr. Pallin was prohibited from enforcing his patent claims on a particular type of incision used in cataract surgery (3). As a result of this case, Congress enacted a 1996 statute making patents of medical or surgical procedures unenforceable (4). In the United States, medical and surgical procedures are still patentable, but patent claims are not enforceable against a medical practitioner unless the practitioner uses a patented pharmaceutical, medical device, or biotechnology process. Thus, the U.S. legal system provides some support for the traditional ethic of physicians to share their knowledge and use of advances in medical and surgical procedures. Other countries view the patentability of medical procedures differently than the United States. For instance, the European Union and Great Britain consider medical procedures to be nonpatentable subject matter.

Patenting Surgical and Diagnostic Instruments

The U.S. patent system also permits medical and surgical devices to be patented, including surgical and diagnostic instruments. The U.S. patent protection permits the patent holder to exclude other individuals or entities from making, using, or selling the patented invention in the United States for a period of 20 years, thus providing market exclusivity to the patent holder. Both ethically and legally, physicians may obtain patents on surgical or diagnostic instruments that they have invented (5). However, out of concern for the welfare of patients, the patent holder should make the instrument available at a fair and reasonable cost.

Patenting Drugs

The granting of patents to pharmaceutical companies for drugs that they have developed may appear to be relatively uncontroversial. Drug makers have successfully argued the need for patent protection to recoup the cost of their investment in drug research and to gain a profit before the makers of generic equivalent drugs are permitted to enter the market.

However, some techniques used by pharmaceutical companies to extend the terms of their patents and their products' market exclusivities have recently come under criticism. For example, companies have paid manufacturers of generic drugs to drop a legal challenge to a patent or to postpone the manufacture of a generic equivalent, they have developed minimally altered formulations or dosages that become eligible for new patents, and they have lobbied Congress for statutory and legislative patent extensions on highly profitable drugs. These techniques may allow the patent holder to continue to charge prices that are far higher than would be the case in a competitive market and to extend the government-sanctioned market exclusivity long beyond when the original patent term would have expired. As a result, the cost to consumers or patients may be inflated beyond providing a reasonable return on research investments and may, in fact, prevent some patients from using drugs that would be beneficial to them. As patients bear an increasing share of the cost of their prescribed drugs, the issue of drug pricing and extended market exclusivities should be of concern to physicians, because it may influence patient compliance with physician recommendations.

The Patenting of Genes

Patent and Trademark Office Guidance

The PTO maintains that genes and gene sequences are patentable subject matter under existing U.S. federal statutes and case law. Since 1980, more than 20,000 patents on genes or other gene-related molecules have been granted, but this total includes gene patents for all organisms, not only humans. More than 25,000 applications for patents on genes or related molecules are pending (6).

Because of continuing controversy over the granting of patents on genes and gene sequences, the PTO has attempted to clarify its standards for granting such patents in its final guidelines on the written description and utility requirements of patents. The guidelines were issued after consideration of public comments on interim guidelines, and they are pertinent to gene patents. The PTO guidelines confirm that an isolated and purified gene (a chemical entity modified from its natural state) is not a naturally occurring substance. Substances as they occur in nature in an unisolated form are not patentable.

Under U.S. patent law, the PTO regards a newly isolated gene or modified gene sequence to be a "composition of matter." This is subject matter that is eligible for a product patent as long as the product satisfies all the statutory conditions for a patent. These conditions require that the patent specification describes an invention that is a new discovery or improvement (novel), that is not obvious to those with ordinary skill in the art (inventive), and that has utility (is useful) (1). Product patents may be enforced broadly against a variety of uses of the claimed product. For example, a product patent claiming an isolated gene sequence can be used to exclude others from using the sequence for commercial purposes (ie, both the isolated gene sequence and the methods of using it in tests and treatments).

If the gene sequence is not new, it may nonetheless be eligible for a use patent (ie, a patent having claims directed to the product's use). The enforcement of a use patent is narrower, being limited to the patented use. Although a use patent restricts the right to use a patented method using a product or composition, it does not restrict access to the product or composition itself.

A patent claiming an isolated gene covers the isolated gene but does not apply to the gene as it occurs in nature. Genes as they occur in the body are not patentable because they do not exist in an isolated and purified form. Therefore, individuals who possess such genes in their bodies would not infringe the patent.

In its final guidelines on the utility requirement for patentability, the PTO requires that the utility be "specific, substantial, and credible" (7). To satisfy this requirement, the inventor must disclose at least one way in which the purified gene, isolated from its natural state, may be used or applied, for example, for diagnostic or predictive genetic testing. However, if the applicant does not explicitly identify a specific utility for the isolated gene sequence, the guidelines permit the utility requirement to be satisfied if the examiner believes that an individual with ordinary skill in the art would recognize that the gene or sequence has a readily apparent "well-established utility." Some commentators have suggested that this well-established utility may be simply a comparison with a structurally analogous gene or sequence that is known to have utility.

In the view of some commentators, the PTO guidelines do not set a high enough standard for establishing the usefulness of a gene or gene sequence and thereby may deem a product useful and allow a patent to be issued covering a gene or gene sequence before the applicant is able to identify a specific practical application (8). Allowing patents on genes and sequences to be issued before their function and purpose are adequately identified could create barriers to other researchers' pursuing such studies or could lessen the incentive for them to do so. Moreover, researchers warn against relying too heavily on structural analogues to predict utility, because minor changes in a gene sequence "may produce profound changes in biological activity" (9).

Gene Patents and the Interests of Patients

Those who support the granting of broad patents believe that patent protection encourages rather than impedes research. It was the intent of Congress that the disclosure required to secure a patent and the limited exclusivity provided by the patent would stimulate progress in science and the useful arts. As the PTO notes, a patent application requires complete public disclosure of the invention, discovery, or improvement and, therefore, may promote dissemination of knowledge rather than secrecy. In the PTO's view, gene patents foster scientific progress because other inventors are encouraged to discover new uses beyond the one specified in the patent application (7). Inventors who develop new and nonobvious uses for a patented gene may patent these inventions, according to the PTO, thereby rewarding researchers who develop the genetic information to the endpoint of a useful method or product (10, 11).

Opponents of broad gene patenting fear that the welfare of the patient, the traditional role of the physician, and the public trust are compromised by gene patents. According to opponents of gene patenting, the patenting of genes can impinge on the interests of patients in at least 4 ways:

1. By retarding the transmission of knowledge (possible if researchers choose to delay the announcement or the publication of their findings until after a patent application is filed)

2. By inhibiting other researchers from pursuing further investigation on the patented product (developing a subsequent invention often is difficult, complicated, or unprofitable because of the need to coordinate licensing with the original patent holder)

3. By establishing a monopoly on all diagnostic and predictive tests based on a patented gene (such action would limit the ability of practitioners and researchers to improve genetic testing by adding new mutations, devising new testing techniques, and developing national quality assurance programs [12])

4. By infringing on the interests of groups of patients who have provided the original genetic material on which the discovery of a gene or sequence is based (they may feel that their concerns are disregarded because of restrictions on access to tests and treatments made possible by their contribution of biologic material)

European challenges to the patent on the breast cancer gene *BRCA1* illustrate problems that arise when a patent holder claims that a patent on a gene precludes other researchers or organizations from developing their own tests for gene mutations. French researchers, supported by the European parliament, argue that such a monopoly could impede or even prevent the development and use of cheaper and more effective tests for *BRCA1* mutations, such as tests that cover a broader range of mutations (13, 14).

Similarly, in the clinical setting, experience has shown that patent holders may in effect deprive patients and physicians of reasonable access (eg, to a genetic test) by placing significant hurdles to its use. These hurdles can include substantial royalties or licensing fees and restrictions on the licensing of clinics or on the number of tests allowed, such as the conditions placed on prenatal and carrier testing for some autosomal recessive diseases (15).

Responses to the problem of restricted access to patented genes have led to several proposed solutions. One proposed solution is to develop a system similar to the music licensing system, where gene patent holders would be required to grant nonexclusive licenses for a reasonable set fee (16). Another

proposed solution is that genes and genetic sequences should not be granted composition-of-matter patents, because the market exclusivity of their patents extends beyond the use identified by the patent applicant and covers uses of the substance that may be discovered later. Instead, a patent would be granted to an applicant who identifies a specific function of a gene, but the patent would cover only the use or utility identified, such as a particular genetic test. Then researchers who later discovered additional applications for the gene would be able to patent these new discoveries (17).

Response to the issue of access to genetic tests has led some patient advocacy groups to take a proactive stance at the time that patients provide tissue samples to researchers. To ensure that any genetic tests that result from their participation will be inexpensive and widely available, these groups are seeking patents held jointly by the patient group and the researchers (18). Therefore, rather than objecting to the patenting of genes and genetic tests, these patients are seeking to use the patent system to protect their own interests.

Recommendations

Practitioners and researchers need to be aware of public policies that may jeopardize their ability to advance medical knowledge and provide the best tests and treatments to patients. Although those who develop useful drugs, diagnostic and screening tests, and medical technologies have the right to expect a fair return for their efforts and risks, current interpretations of patent law have the potential to impede rather than promote scientific and medical advances. Because the purpose of the patent system is to promote the public welfare, practices that are inimical to the public good and overly protective of commercial monopolies should be altered (17).

Policies regarding the patenting of scientific inventions, discoveries, and improvements must balance the need for the open exchange and use of information with the need to make the pursuit of such knowledge financially rewarding. Therefore, the Committee on Ethics and the Committee on Genetics of the American College of Obstetricians and Gynecologists suggest the following recommendations regarding the patenting of medical and surgical procedures, medical devices, genes, DNA sequences, screening and diagnostic tests, and gene-based therapies:

1. Patents on medical or surgical procedures are ethically unacceptable, and some are legally

unenforceable. Physicians may obtain patents on surgical and diagnostic instruments that they have developed. However, the patent holders should make these instruments available at a fair and reasonable cost for the benefit of patients.

2. Because a patent claiming a gene as a composition of matter enables a patent holder to control future applications of the patented gene or sequence, such patents should not be granted. A patent should be granted only for the specified use or application of the gene or sequence (a "use" patent), thus enabling others to develop additional applications (17). Because case law and the PTO interpret a gene as being a patentable chemical composition of matter, such a limitation would require congressional intervention. The Committee on Ethics and the Committee on Genetics support legislation that would make composition-of-matter patents on genes unenforceable.

3. If composition-of-matter patents on genes continue to be enforceable, such patents on genes with clinical applications should be subject to federal regulation and oversight to ensure reasonable availability of the genes and their products for research and clinical use. Such regulation should include requirements on licensing arrangements to ensure access for the public good, including both the advancement of knowledge and the clinical care of patients. Specifically, licensing agreements should permit reasonable but not excessive royalties and should allow unlimited access to tests by qualified laboratories, precluding exclusionary arrangements and quotas on the number of tests that may be offered.

References

1. 35 U.S.C. §101–103, 112 (2001).
2. American Medical Association Council on Ethical and Judicial Affairs. Code of medical ethics: current opinions with annotations. Chicago (IL): AMA; 2002. p. 263–4.
3. Pallin v. Singer 1995 U.S. Dist. LEXIS 20824, 36 U.S.P.Q2d (BNA) 1050 (D.Vt. May 1 1995).
4. Patents and Protection of Patent Rights: Remedies for Infringement of Patent and Other Actions, 35 U.S.C. 287(c)(1) (2001).
5. American Medical Association Council on Ethical and Judicial Affairs. Code of medical ethics: current opinions with annotations. Chicago (IL): AMA; 2002. p. 262–3.
6. Doll JJ. Talking gene patents. Sci Am 2001;285:28.
7. Utility examination guidelines. Fed Regist 2001;66: 1092–9.
8. Public comments on guidelines for determining utility of gene-related patents. Released by U.S. Patent and Trademark Office, April 19, 2000. Available at http://www.uspto.gov/web/offices/com/sol/comments/utilguide/index.html. Retrieved May 22, 2002.
9. Spiegel J. Comment 44. 2000. Available at http://www.uspto.gov/web/offices/com/sol/comments/utilguide/nih2.pdf. Retrieved June 28, 2002.
10. Doll JJ. The patenting of DNA. Science 1998;280:689–90.
11. Wheeler DL. Will DNA patents hinder research? Lawyers say not to worry. Chronicle of Higher Education, July 16, 1999, p. A19.
12. American College of Medical Genetics. Position statement on gene patents and accessibility of gene testing. 1999. Available at http://www.faseb.org/genetics/acmg/pol-34.htm. Retrieved June 10, 2002.
13. Dorozynski A. France challenges patent for genetic screening of breast cancer. BMJ 2001;323:589.
14. Watson R. MEPs protest at patent for breast cancer gene. BMJ 2001;323:888.
15. Marshall E. Genetic testing. Families sue hospital, scientist for control of Canavan gene. Science 2000;290:1062.
16. Heller MA, Eisenberg RS. Can patents deter innovation? The anticommons in biomedical research. Science 1998; 280:698–701.
17. Williamson AR. Gene patents: socially acceptable monopolies or an unnecessary hindrance to research? Trends Genet 2001;17:670–3.
18. Smaglik P. Tissue donors use their influence in deal over gene patent terms. Nature 2000;407:821.

Suggested Reading

U.S. Department of Energy Office of Science. Genetics and Patenting. 2002. Available at http://www.ornl.gov/hgmis/elsi/patents.html. Retrieved June 28, 2002.

United States Patent and Trademark Office. General information concerning patents. 2002. Available at http://www.uspto.gov/web/offices/pac/doc/general/index.html. Retrieved June 28, 2002.

Expert Testimony

The American College of Obstetricians and Gynecologists (ACOG) recognizes that it is the duty of obstetricians and gynecologists who testify as expert witnesses on behalf of defendants, the government, or plaintiffs to do so solely in accordance with their judgment on the merits of the case. Furthermore, ACOG cannot condone the participation of physicians in legal actions where their testimony will impugn performance that falls within accepted standards of practice or, conversely, will support obviously deficient practice. Because the experts articulate the standards in a given case, care must be exercised to ensure that such standards do not narrowly reflect the experts' views to the exclusion of other choices deemed acceptable by the profession. The American College of Obstetricians and Gynecologists considers unethical any expert testimony that is misleading because the witness does not have appropriate knowledge of the standard of care for the particular condition at the relevant time or because the witness knowingly misrepresents the standard of care relevant to the case.

The Problem of Professional Liability— Reality and Perceptions

The American College of Obstetricians and Gynecologists recognizes its responsibility, and that of its Fellows, to continue efforts to improve health care for women through every available method of quality assurance. The American College of Obstetricians and Gynecologists also recognizes, however, that many claims of medical malpractice represent the response of a litigation-oriented society to a technologically advanced form of health

care that has fostered unrealistic expectations. As technology continues to become more complex, both the benefits and risks also increase, making the complication-free practice of medicine less possible.

It therefore becomes important to distinguish between medical "maloccurrence" and medical malpractice. Medical maloccurrence is defined as a bad outcome that is unrelated to the quality of care provided. Certain medical or surgical complications can be anticipated and represent unavoidable risks of appropriate medical care. Other complications arise unpredictably and are similarly unavoidable. Still others occur as a result of decisions that have been made carefully by patients and physicians with fully informed consent but appear, in retrospect, to have been a less appropriate choice among several options. Each of these situations represents a type of maloccurrence, rather than an example of malpractice, and is the result of the uncertainty inherent in all of medicine. Malpractice requires a demonstration of negligence (ie, substandard practice that causes harm). The potential for personal, professional, and financial rewards from expert testimony may encourage testimony that undermines the distinction between unavoidable maloccurrence and actual medical malpractice. It is unethical to distort or to represent a maloccurrence as an example of medical malpractice, or the converse.

The American College of Obstetricians and Gynecologists supports the concept of appropriate and prompt compensation to patients for medically related injuries. Any such response, however, also should reflect the distinction between medical maloccurrence, for which all of society should perhaps bear financial responsibility, and medical malpractice, for which health care providers should be held responsible.

Previously published as Committee Opinion 217, April 1999; content revised January 2004

Responsibility of Individual Physicians

The moral and legal duty of physicians who testify before a court of law is to do so in accordance with their expertise. This duty implies adherence to the strictest personal and professional ethics. Truthfulness is essential. Misrepresentation of one's personal clinical opinion as absolute right or wrong may be harmful to individual parties and to the profession at large. The obstetrician–gynecologist who is an expert witness must limit testimony to his or her sphere of medical expertise and must be prepared adequately. Witnesses who testify as experts must have knowledge and experience that are relevant to obstetric and gynecologic practice at the time of the occurrence and to the specific areas of clinical medicine they are discussing. The acceptance of fees that are greatly disproportionate to those customary for professional services can be construed as influencing testimony given by the witness. It is unethical for a physician to accept compensation that is contingent on the outcome of litigation (1, 2).

The American College of Obstetricians and Gynecologists encourages the development of policies and standards for expert testimony. Such policies should address safeguards to promote truth-telling and to encourage openness of the testimony to peer review. These policies also would encourage testimony that does not assume an advocacy or partisan role in the legal proceeding.

The following principles are offered as guidelines for the physician who assumes the role of an expert witness:

1. The physician must have experience and knowledge in the areas of clinical medicine that enable him or her to testify about the standards of care that applied at the time of the occurrence that is the subject of the legal action.

2. The physician's review of medical facts must be thorough, fair, and impartial and must not exclude any relevant information. It must not be biased to create a view favoring the plaintiff, the government, or the defendant. The goal of a physician testifying in any judicial proceeding should be to provide testimony that is complete, objective, and helpful to a just resolution of the proceeding.

3. The physician's testimony must reflect an evaluation of performance in light of generally accepted standards, neither condemning performance that falls within generally accepted practice standards nor endorsing or condoning performance that falls below these standards. Medical decisions often must be made in the absence of diagnostic and prognostic certainty.

4. The physician must make a clear distinction between medical malpractice and medical maloccurrence.

5. The physician must make every effort to assess the relationship of the alleged substandard practice to the outcome, because deviation from a practice standard is not always substandard care or causally related to a bad outcome.

6. The physician must be prepared to have testimony given in any judicial proceeding subjected to peer review by an institution or professional organization to which he or she belongs.

References

1. American Medical Association. Medical testimony. In: Code of medical ethics: current opinions with annotations. Chicago (IL): AMA; 2002. p. 259–61.
2. American Bar Association. Rule 3.4 Fairness to opposing party and counsel. Annotated model rules of professional conduct. 5th ed. Chicago (IL): ABA; 2003. p. 347–58.

Code of Professional Ethics
of the American College of
Obstetricians and Gynecologists

Obstetrician–gynecologists, as members of the medical profession, have ethical responsibilities not only to patients, but also to society, to other health professionals, and to themselves. The following ethical foundations for professional activities in the field of obstetrics and gynecology are the supporting structures for the Code of Conduct. The Code implements many of these foundations in the form of rules of ethical conduct. Certain documents of the American College of Obstetricians and Gynecologists, including Committee Opinions and *Ethics in Obstetrics and Gynecology*, also provide additional ethical rules. Selections relevant to specific points are set forth in the Code of Conduct, and those particular documents are incorporated into the Code by reference. Noncompliance with the Code, including referenced documents, may affect an individual's initial or continuing Fellowship in the American College of Obstetricians and Gynecologists. These documents may be revised or replaced periodically, and Fellows should be knowledgeable about current information.

Ethical Foundations

I. The patient–physician relationship: The welfare of the patient *(beneficence)* is central to all considerations in the patient–physician relationship. Included in this relationship is the obligation of physicians to respect the rights of patients, colleagues, and other health professionals. The respect for the right of individual patients to make their own choices about their health care *(autonomy)* is fundamental. The principle of justice requires strict avoidance of discrimination on the basis of race, color, religion, national origin, or any other basis that would constitute illegal discrimination *(justice)*.

II.   Physician conduct and practice: The obstetrician–gynecologist must deal honestly with patients and colleagues *(veracity)*. This includes not misrepresenting himself or herself through any form of communication in an untruthful, misleading, or deceptive manner. Furthermore, maintenance of medical competence through study, application, and enhancement of medical knowledge and skills is an obligation of practicing physicians. Any behavior that diminishes a physician's capability to practice, such as substance abuse, must be immediately addressed and rehabilitative services instituted. The physician should modify his or her practice until the diminished capacity has been restored to an acceptable standard to avoid harm to patients *(nonmaleficence)*. All physicians are obligated to respond to evidence of questionable conduct or unethical behavior by other physicians through appropriate procedures established by the relevant organization.

III. Avoiding conflicts of interest: Potential conflicts of interest are inherent in the practice of medicine. Physicians are expected to recognize such situations and deal with them through public disclosure. Conflicts of interest should be resolved in accordance with the best interest of the patient, respecting a woman's autonomy to make health care decisions. The physician should be an advocate for the patient through public disclosure of conflicts of interest raised by health payer policies or hospital policies.

IV.   Professional relations: The obstetrician–gynecologist should respect and cooperate with other physicians, nurses, and health care professionals.

V.   Societal responsibilities: The obstetrician–gynecologist has a continuing responsibility to society as a whole and should support and participate in activities that enhance the community. As a member of society, the obstetrician–gynecologist should respect the laws of that society. As professionals and members of medical societies, physicians are required to uphold the dignity and honor of the profession.

Code of Conduct

I.   Patient–Physician Relationship

1. The patient–physician relationship is the central focus of all ethical concerns, and the welfare of the patient must form the basis of all medical judgments.

2. The obstetrician–gynecologist should serve as the patient's advocate and exercise all reasonable means to ensure that the most appropriate care is provided to the patient.

3. The patient–physician relationship has an ethical basis and is built on confidentiality, trust, and honesty. If no patient–physician relationship exists, a physician may refuse to provide care, except in emergencies (1). Once the patient–physician relationship exists, the obstetrician–gynecologist must adhere to all applicable legal or contractual constraints in dissolving the patient–physician relationship.

4. Sexual misconduct on the part of the obstetrician–gynecologist is an abuse of professional power and a violation of patient trust. Sexual contact or a romantic relationship between a physician and a current patient is always unethical (2).

5. The obstetrician–gynecologist has an obligation to obtain the informed consent of each patient (3). In obtaining informed consent for any course of medical or surgical treatment, the obstetrician–gynecologist must present to the patient, or to the person legally responsible for the patient, pertinent medical facts and recommendations consistent with good medical practice. Such information should be presented in reasonably understandable terms and include alternative modes of treatment and the objectives, risks, benefits, possible complications, and anticipated results of such treatment.

6. It is unethical to prescribe, provide, or seek compensation for therapies that are of no benefit to the patient.

7. The obstetrician–gynecologist must respect the rights and privacy of patients, colleagues, and others and safeguard patient information and confidences within the limits of the law. If during the process of providing information for consent it is known that results of a particular test or other information must be given to governmental authorities or other third parties, that must be explained to the patient (4).

8. The obstetrician–gynecologist must not discriminate against patients based on race, color, national origin, religion, or any other basis that would constitute illegal discrimination.

II. Physician Conduct and Practice

1. The obstetrician–gynecologist should recognize the boundaries of his or her particular competencies and expertise and must provide only those services and use only those techniques for which he or she is qualified by education, training, and experience.

2. The obstetrician–gynecologist should participate in continuing medical education activities to maintain current scientific and professional knowledge relevant to the medical services he or she renders. The obstetrician–gynecologist should provide medical care involving new therapies or techniques only after undertaking appropriate training and study.

3. In emerging areas of medical treatment where recognized medical guidelines do not exist, the obstetrician–gynecologist should exercise careful judgment and take appropriate precautions to protect patient welfare.

4. The obstetrician–gynecologist must not publicize or represent himself or herself in any untruthful, misleading, or deceptive manner to patients, colleagues, other health care professionals, or the public.

5. The obstetrician–gynecologist who has reason to believe that he or she is infected with the human immunodeficiency virus (HIV) or other serious infectious agents that might be communicated to patients should voluntarily be tested for the protection of his or her patients. In making decisions about patient-care activities, a physician infected with such an agent should adhere to the fundamental professional obligation to avoid harm to patients (5).

6. The obstetrician–gynecologist should not practice medicine while impaired by alcohol, drugs, or physical or mental disability. The obstetrician–gynecologist who experiences substance abuse problems or who is physically or emotionally impaired should seek appropriate assistance to address these problems and must limit his or her practice until the impairment no longer affects the quality of patient care.

III. Conflicts of Interest

1. Potential conflicts of interest are inherent in the practice of medicine. Conflicts of interest should be resolved in accordance with the best interest of the patient, respecting a woman's autonomy to make health care decisions. If there is an actual or potential conflict of interest that could be reasonably construed to affect significantly the patient's care, the physician must disclose the conflict to the patient. The physician should seek consultation with colleagues or an institutional ethics committee to determine whether there is an actual or potential conflict of interest and how to address it.

2. Commercial promotions of medical products and services may generate bias unrelated to product merit, creating or appearing to create inappropriate undue influence. The obstetrician–gynecologist should be aware of this potential conflict of interest and offer medical advice that is as accurate, balanced, complete, and devoid of bias as possible (6, 7).

3. The obstetrician–gynecologist should prescribe drugs, devices, and other treatments solely on the basis of medical considerations and patient needs, regardless of any direct or indirect interests in or benefit from a pharmaceutical firm or other supplier.

4. When the obstetrician–gynecologist receives anything of substantial value, including royalties, from companies in the health care industry, such as a manufacturer of pharmaceuticals and medical devices, this fact should be disclosed to patients and colleagues when material.

5. Financial and administrative constraints may create disincentives to treatment otherwise recommended by the obstetrician–gynecologist. Any pertinent constraints should be disclosed to the patient.

IV. Professional Relations

1. The obstetrician–gynecologist's relationships with other physicians, nurses, and health care professionals should reflect fairness, honesty, and integrity, sharing a mutual respect and concern for the patient.

2. The obstetrician–gynecologist should consult, refer, or cooperate with other physicians, health care professionals, and institutions to the extent necessary to serve the best interests of their patients.

V. Societal Responsibilities

1. The obstetrician–gynecologist should support and participate in those health care programs, practices, and activities that contribute positively, in a meaningful and cost-effective way, to the welfare of individual patients, the health care system, or the public good.

2. The obstetrician–gynecologist should respect all laws, uphold the dignity and honor of the profession, and accept the profession's self-imposed discipline. The professional competence and conduct of obstetrician–gynecologists are best examined by professional associations, hospital peer-review committees, and state medical and licensing boards. These groups deserve the full participation and cooperation of the obstetrician–gynecologist.

3. The obstetrician–gynecologist should strive to address through the appropriate procedures the status of those physicians who demonstrate questionable competence, impairment, or unethical or illegal behavior. In addition, the obstetrician–gynecologist should cooperate with appropriate authorities to prevent the continuation of such behavior.

4. The obstetrician–gynecologist must not knowingly offer testimony that is false. The obstetrician–gynecologist must testify only on matters about which he or she has knowledge and experience. The obstetrician–gynecologist must not knowingly misrepresent his or her credentials.

5. The obstetrician–gynecologist testifying as an expert witness must have knowledge and experience about the range of the standard of care and the available scientific evidence for the condition in question during the relevant time and must respond accurately to questions about the range of the standard of care and the available scientific evidence.

6. Before offering testimony, the obstetrician–gynecologist must thoroughly review the medical facts of the case and all available relevant information.

7. The obstetrician–gynecologist serving as an expert witness must accept neither disproportionate compensation nor compensation that is contingent upon the outcome of the litigation (8).

References

1. American College of Obstetricians and Gynecologists. Seeking and giving consultation. In: Ethics in obstetrics and gynecology. 2nd ed. Washington, DC: ACOG; 2004. p. 77–81.

2. American College of Obstetricians and Gynecologists. Sexual misconduct. In: Ethics in obstetrics and gynecology. 2nd ed. Washington, DC: ACOG; 2004. p. 101–3.

3. American College of Obstetricians and Gynecologists. Informed consent. In: Ethics in obstetrics and gynecology. 2nd ed. Washington, DC: ACOG; 2004. p. 9–17.

4. American College of Obstetricians and Gynecologists. Patient testing. In: Ethics in obstetrics and gynecology. 2nd ed. Washington, DC: ACOG; 2004. p. 26–8.

5. American College of Obstetricians and Gynecologists. Human immunodeficiency virus. In: Ethics in obstetrics and gynecology. 2nd ed. Washington, DC: ACOG; 2004. p. 29–33.

6. American College of Obstetricians and Gynecologists. Relationships with industry. In: Ethics in obstetrics and gynecology. 2nd ed. Washington, DC: ACOG; 2004. p. 107–10.

7. American College of Obstetricians and Gynecologists. Commercial enterprises in medical practice. In: Ethics in obstetrics and gynecology. 2nd ed. Washington, DC: ACOG; 2004. p. 83–5.

8. American College of Obstetricians and Gynecologists. Expert testimony. In: Ethics in obstetrics and gynecology. 2nd ed. Washington, DC: ACOG; 2004. p. 116–7.

Index